Diagnostic Laryngology

Adults & Children

**BRUCE N.P. BENJAMIN,
O.B.E., F.R.A.C.S, D.L.O.**

Lecturer in Diseases of the Ear, Nose, and Throat.
The William Blano Center
Sydney, Australia

1990
W. B. SAUNDERS COMPANY
Harcourt Brace Jovanovich, Inc
Philadelphia · London · Toronto · Montreal · Sydney · Tokyo

W. B. SAUNDERS COMPANY
Harcourt Brace Jovanovich, Inc.

The Curtis Center
Independence Square West
Philadelphia, PA 19106

Library of Congress Cataloging-in-Publication Data

Benjamin, Bruce.
    Diagnostic Laryngology: Adults and Children/Bruce N.P. Benjamin.
        p.   cm.
        1. Laryngoscopy—Atlases.   2. Larynx—Radiography—Atlases.
    3. Pediatric otolaryngology—Atlases.   I. Title.
        [DNLM: 1. Laryngeal Diseases—diagnosis—atlases.
    2. Laryngoscopy—atlases.   WV 17 B468a]
    RF514.B45 1990
    616.2′2075—dc20
    DNLM/DLC   89-6212
        ISBN 0-7216-2838-9

Designer: Terri Siegel

Production Manager: Bob Butler

Manuscript Editor: Mark Coyle

Illustration Coordinator: Peg Shaw

Indexer: Susan Thomas

Cover Designer: Michelle Maloney

ISBN 0-7216-2838-9
Diagnostic Laryngology: Adults and Children

Printed in the United States

Last digit is the print number: 9   8   7   6   5   4   3   2   1

To my wife Nellie, son Gregory,
and daughter Susanne for their
steadfast support

Preface

This book is about endoscopic diagnosis of laryngeal disease. It is a comprehensive guide to diseases as they are seen at direct endoscopy using general anesthesia and describes endoscopic techniques for the larynx in adults and for the larynx and upper airways in infants and children. Accurate diagnosis is the basis of logical, rational management. Documentation by endoscopic photographs and x-rays provides a reference for diagnosis and understanding of problems that confront the otolaryngologist, endoscopist, and anesthesiologist. Color photography during direct endoscopic examination with the patient under general anesthesia is the best method of documentation for case management or for publication in printed form, while endoscopic video recording, although more complicated and expensive, is best for study of laryngeal dynamics.

Kleinsasser introduced and popularized microlaryngoscopy in the 1960's, and after his text *Microlaryngoscopy and Endolaryngeal Microsurgery* a new era in laryngology blossomed. The operating microscope, familiar to otologists for many years, is now used universally for microsurgery of the larynx. Specially designed operating laryngoscopes for microsurgery can be fixed in position by a self-retaining laryngoscope holder, but this method of suspension laryngoscopy somewhat limits manipulation and restricts visualization. The application of an additional technique is described in this book; it requires preliminary naked eye examination with a hand-held laryngoscope followed by a more detailed evaluation using rigid telescopes for image magnification. Angled telescopes are utilized for examination of the laryngeal ventricles, the anterior and posterior commissure, and the subglottic region and beyond obstructive lesions. Telescopes are a more convenient means of performing a thorough diagnostic examination, and they facilitate routine photographic documentation.

A survey of the oropharynx and laryngopharynx with a suitable hand-held laryngoscope and rigid telescopes precedes and is combined with the microlaryngeal technique when endolaryngeal surgery is required. A comprehensive evaluation of the upper airway and larynx using these techniques will be outlined together with the equipment and techniques that have become standard. As almost all endoscopic examinations are performed with the use of general anesthesia, the modern, controlled, and safe anesthetic techniques employed will be reviewed.

I wish to thank my colleagues in anesthesia at Sydney Hospital, Royal North Shore Hospital, and the Royal Alexandra Hospital for Children. Without their skill, collaboration, patience, and enthusiasm, this work would not have been possible. Karl Storz has been consistently helpful with research and development of instruments. John Collins, medical artist, together with Pixie Maloney and Reg Money, medical photographers, have given their skilled professional support over many years.

Foreword

Throughout the history of otolaryngology (laryngology and bronchoesophagology in particular), the quality that has characterized our greatest scientists and educators has been the ability to demonstrate the principles of anatomy and pathology through illustrations. As a youth, Chevalier Jackson established his skills as an artist, supplementing the meager income of a coal miner's family by painting birds and flowers on china cups. Later, at his well known "chalk talks," he rapidly and bimanually drew detailed illustrations of laryngeal anatomy and pathology.

The particular problem that faces the endoscopist is illustrating an operative field that may measure no more than a few millimeters in diameter. It is difficult enough to recognize pathology in such a small field, but to demonstrate this for others is even more difficult. The first good-quality endoscopic color photography was presented in 1946 by Paul H. Holinger, M.D., in his Thesis for the Casselberry Award of the American Laryngological Association. At last the larynx could be viewed by projected lantern slides on a screen 6 feet in diameter before an audience of several hundred. The Holinger-Brubaker endoscopic camera, developed in conjunction with the photographic engineer Joseph Brubaker, made this possible.

Paul Ward, George Berci, Eiji Yanagigisawa, and Bruce Benjamin have set the standard for the most recent generation of endoscopic photography using Hopkins rod-lens telescopes with fiber illumination. Of these, Bruce Benjamin has excelled in endoscopic photography of the infant and child. His previous book, *Atlas of Paediatric Endoscopy: Upper Respiratory Tract and Oesophagus*, has become a standard by which all other similar endeavors are measured. With this new book the author has extended his expertise to an audience that includes all otolaryngologists. His work is truly an embodiment of the ancient proverb: "One showing is worth a thousand times talking about."

In addition to the superb color endoscopic photographs, the first part of the text is illustrated with the black and white line drawings of Mr. John Collins from the Department of Medical Illustration at the Sydney Hospital. Mr. Collins has collaborated with the author in the past, and the sure and clear strokes of his pen precisely take form to dramatize the point the author wishes to convey to the reader.

Bruce Benjamin is the consummate otolaryngologist for all seasons, traveling the Southern and Northern hemispheres with great frequency from his native Australia. His experience as a pediatric otolaryngologist, and endoscopist in particular, has achieved worldwide recognition. He regularly brings to international meetings fresh and creative approaches for old and difficult problems, and his presentations are all superbly illustrated, as one would anticipate from a careful inspection of this book. His many talents include the development of new instruments and techniques and the education of students, residents, and fellows.

This volume serves as a testimony to the success of Bruce Benjamin's illustrious career. It provides a practical and dramatic perspective of the human larynx to the novice and the experienced surgeon alike. It is eminently successful as a work of art, a scientific endeavor, and a superb teaching medium.

LAUREN D. HOLINGER, M.D.
Chicago

Contents

PART ONE

Indications and Techniques

PRESENTING FEATURES

Adults

The cardinal feature of laryngeal disease in adults is an alteration in the voice. The voice may be husky (relentlessly progressive with malignancy, persistent with multiple papilloma, variable with vocal nodules), weak (unilateral vocal cord paralysis), breathy (hysterical dysphonia), strained and choking (spastic dysphonia), high-pitched (falsetto after adolescence), or dysarthyric (neurological disease).

These changes in phonation are related to airflow and pressure from the lower respiratory tract, tension and mass of the vocal folds, neurological control of vocal cord movement, alteration of movement of one or both vocal folds, and changes of vocal fold tension and vibration.

In adults certain objective methods of study of voice disorders can be applied when patients are studied in a fully equipped voice laboratory. These techniques include studies of airflow, maximum phonation time, subglottic air pressure, high-speed cinephotography, video-fluoroscopy, electromyography, phonoglottography, and video recording with flexible fiberoptics. Stroboscopy and strobovideolaryngoscopy permit assessment of the pattern of vocal cord vibration but are expensive and unlikely to be used universally. Further study of these techniques is beyond the scope of this book.

Further information about the history of the clinical features is necessary to correlate the description, duration, and nature of the symptoms with the physical findings. For instance, there are certain features with regard to hoarseness.

HOARSENESS

Onset. Sudden onset while shouting is likely to be due to hemorrhage into a vocal cord, whereas sudden onset following a thyroid operation is likely to be due to damage to one or even both recurrent laryngeal nerves.

Duration. Hoarseness lasting a few days following an upper respiratory tract infection is likely to be due to acute inflammatory laryngitis, whereas huskiness for many years could be due to Reinke's edema.

Progression. Relentless progression of symptoms strongly suggests a neoplastic cause.

Variability. Huskiness caused by vocal nodules is always present but can vary in severity depending upon overuse, misuse, or abuse of the voice. Voice abnormality as an early manifestation of neurological disease might at first be variable and irregular.

OTHER CLINICAL FEATURES

Other important presenting symptoms include a feeling of "something in the throat," pain referred to the ear, difficulty swallowing, or the presence of a lump in the neck.

3

Infants and Children

Whereas hoarseness is the cardinal symptom of laryngeal pathology in adults, stridor is the foremost feature of upper airway disease in infants and children. Stridor is an abnormal sound due to partial obstruction of the upper airway, including the laryngeal airway. The stridor is usually inspiratory, sometimes expiratory, and occasionally both inspiratory and expiratory. It is heard by listening while beside the patient, whereas a wheeze, such as the expiratory accompaniment of asthma, is heard by auscultation with a stethoscope. It is necessary to know when the stridor commenced; how long it has been present; whether it is acute or chronic; what has been the progression, variability, and severity; the relationship to inspiration and expiration; and the effect of sleeping, feeding, crying, posture, and head position. Observation and examination over a period of hours or days may give useful information not detectable at a single examination, and when time permits such information should be obtained. The characteristics of the stridor are seldom diagnostic in any particular disease. Although it may be possible to make a preliminary diagnosis before endoscopy, direct examination of the nasal cavities, pharynx, larynx, and tracheobronchial tree with the patient under general anesthesia is often necessary to make an exact and final diagnosis. In infants and children it is not possible to study laryngeal disease alone without consideration of the upper airways from the nasal cavities down to the main bronchi.

Pediatric patients with airway problems present for endoscopic assessment with one or more of the following features:

- "Congenital laryngeal stridor"
- Obstruction in the newborn baby
- Acute inflammatory obstruction
- Chronic progressive obstruction
- Croup, recurrent or atypical
- Husky voice
- Inhaled foreign body
- Weak or absent cry
- Repeated aspiration
- Cyanotic attacks
- Apneic attacks
- "Pneumonia" or "bronchitis"
- Tracheobronchial compression
- Mediastinal mass

"Congenital laryngeal stridor" is an unfortunate term. It is no more a diagnosis than "anemia." The cause of the stridor may not be congenital, nor is the stridor necessarily generated from the region of the larynx; it may be due to pharyngeal obstruction by a cyst in the laryngopharynx or tongue, stenosis of the trachea, or a vascular ring causing tracheobronchial compression. Laryngoscopy alone, without examination of the tracheobronchial tree and (in selected cases) the esophagus, must be regarded as an incomplete investigation.

Repeated aspiration in infants requires investigation for incoordinate swallowing, gastroesophageal reflux, H-type tracheoesophageal fistula, or a posterior cleft of the larynx. A mediastinal mass may produce areas of obstructive emphysema or atelectasis and is usually seen on a chest radiograph or on a computed tomography (CT) scan.

Some patients may have symptoms relating to both the airway and the esophagus, for example, tracheoesophageal fistula with esophageal atresia. Finally, each patient must, of course, be evaluated individually. Babies with mild stridor and no respiratory distress may require only observation at regular intervals. Further investigation, including endoscopy, is certainly indicated for:

- Severe stridor
- Progressive stridor
- Stridor associated with unusual features such as cyanotic or apneic attacks, dysphagia, aspiration, or failure to thrive
- A radiological abnormality
- Stridor where there is undue parental anxiety

INDIRECT LARYNGOSCOPY

Mirror Laryngoscopy

Indirect examination of the larynx using a mirror in the oropharynx is the simplest and yet the most helpful diagnostic examination. The appearance of the laryngopharyngeal structures and the movement of the vocal cords can be assessed in adults and in most children over the age of 6 or 7 years.

The examination requires inexpensive equipment but requires a greater than average degree of practiced dexterity. An inexpert or hurried approach makes a relatively easy procedure seem difficult. To provide the best exposure the patient should sit erect with the head slightly forward and the chin up. Adequate illumination, using either a head mirror or a headlight, is essential to reflect a bright beam on the laryngeal mirror. The protruded tongue is held gently but firmly and a suitable-sized mirror, warmed to prevent fogging, is slowly and gently introduced into the oropharynx to avoid touching either the posterior part of the tongue or the posterior pharyngeal wall. The mirror slowly presses the uvula and soft palate upward and backward in a smooth movement to reveal the reflected image of the larynx as the patient breathes quietly and regularly through the mouth. The larynx moves upward and is seen more prominently when the patient phonates a high-pitched sound. The appearance and movement of the laryngeal structures and the vocal cords can then be assessed. Occasionally topical anesthesia is required for patients with a sensitive gag reflex.

Flexible Fiberoptic Laryngoscopy

In some patients, for example, those in whom mirror laryngoscopy even after local anesthesia is not satisfactory, those in whom the mouth cannot be satisfactorily opened, and some children, use of the flexible fiberoptic laryngoscope can yield valuable information that is otherwise unobtainable without general anesthesia. Present-day instruments give an improved image and are usually easy to use. Some patients tolerate passage of the instrument through the nose and oropharynx without topical anesthesia, whereas others need surface anesthesia.

The flexible fiberoptic laryngoscope is introduced through one nasal cavity, guided around the soft palate and behind the base of the tongue and the epiglottis, and positioned to observe the pharyngeal, supraglottic, and glottic structures with particular attention to the appearance and movement of the vocal cords. This method allows visualization of the vocal cords during speech. Because of the flexible fiberoptic threads the image is not as sharp and clear as with a mirror or with a rigid fiberoptic telescope and cannot be considered reliable for the diagnosis of small lesions or early changes.

6

Rigid Telescope Laryngoscopy

A third method of indirect laryngoscopy involves the use of an angled, rigid fiberoptic telescope, with or without a device for focusing and changing the image size. Patients whose gag reflex cannot tolerate the instrument in the oropharynx often require topical analgesia. The view of the larynx and pharynx is excellent, sometimes even better than with a laryngeal mirror.

THE PATIENT'S VOICE

One of the most important elements of the physical examination is evaluation by the laryngologist of the characteristics of the patient's voice. There is no finer instrument for this assessment than the human ear.

INDICATIONS FOR ENDOSCOPY

Indirect laryngoscopy is the fundamental examination for laryngeal diagnosis; however, in some patients it does not provide sufficient information for a complete diagnosis, and direct laryngeal examination becomes necessary. There are many indications for direct laryngoscopy.

Adults

1. Diagnostic examination. In those patients in whom indirect examination has been incomplete or impossible because of difficult anatomy or unduly sensitive reflexes, a symptom such as persistent hoarseness will require direct laryngoscopic diagnostic evaluation with use of anesthesia. Modern anesthetic methods allow assessment of vocal cord movement as muscular tone returns at the end of the procedure.
2. Biopsy of a suspected neoplasm or an unusual mass.
3. Removal of a vocal nodule, polyp, granuloma, Reinke's edema, organized hematoma, or other similar lesion.
4. Laser treatment of multiple papillomas, mucosal dysplasia, early malignancy, and so forth.
5. Teflon or Gelfoam paste injection for a paralyzed vocal cord.
6. Assessment of laryngeal trauma caused by prolonged endotracheal intubation.
7. Treatment of acquired web or stenosis, including endoscopic placement of a stent or keel.
8. Endoscopic arytenoidectomy.

Infants and Children

1. Diagnostic examination to determine the cause of stridor includes direct endoscopic examination of the oropharynx, larynx, and tracheobronchial tree and in selected cases also the esophagus, nasal cavities, and nasopharynx.
2. Investigation of atypical or recurrent croup, a weak or absent cry or a husky voice, repeated aspiration, and so on.
3. Intubation to relieve acute inflammatory airway obstruction caused by severe croup or acute epiglottitis.
4. Removal of an inhaled foreign body in the tracheobronchial tree or the larynx.
5. Assessment of laryngeal trauma caused by prolonged endotracheal intubation.
6. Assessment of tracheobronchial narrowing, collapse, or compression.
7. Laser treatment of lesions such as multiple respiratory papillomas, hemangioma, or lymphangioma.

8. Treatment of congenital or acquired web or stenosis.
9. Pre- or postoperative assessment in infants with tracheoesophageal fistula and esophageal atresia.
10. Endoscopic arytenoidectomy, treatment of congenital subglottic hemangioma, or repair of minor posterior congenital cleft larynx.

RADIOLOGIC EXAMINATION

Imaging techniques utilized to study the larynx and upper airways include conventional plain x-ray and xeroradiogram of the upper airways, chest x-ray, positive-contrast laryngography, coronal tomography, axial CT scan, and magnetic resonance imaging (MRI) studies. Radiography shows the site and sometimes the nature of tumors, provides information for the assessment of soft tissue or pharyngeal space infections, impacted foreign body, cysts, laryngoceles, and congenital abnormalities, and is useful in determining the length and thickness of a stenotic area. Advanced organ imaging, including examination by MRI, helps in defining the pre-epiglottic space, the paralaryngeal spaces, and the laryngeal and tracheal framework. This is particularly useful in laryngeal trauma and in cancer for precise assessment of the suitability for radiation therapy or conservation surgery.

Evidence from the history, the findings on physical examination, and indirect laryngoscopic examination determine the need for further special studies. Radiological studies should always be considered in the investigation of an infant or child with suspected airway difficulty; in some cases it contributes vital information for complete assessment and for planning treatment.

Positive-contrast laryngography was formerly used in adults to show tumor site and size, mucosal irregularities, vocal cord fixation, and thickness of stenotic areas. Other modalities have superseded the laryngogram, and it should no longer be used; an already narrowed airway may be further compromised by introduction of the contrast material.

Soft Tissue Radiography

A lateral view using conventional x-ray or, in selected cases, xeroradiography or high-kilovoltage (Kv) radiography delineates the upper airway (see Figures 50 to 53). A well-exposed film with the head and neck in the hyperextended position often gives information of essential diagnostic value. A high Kv film in the anteroposterior plane enhances the tracheal air column by de-emphasizing the bony cervical spine. Xeroradiography employing a selenium-coated plate enhances the air–soft tissue interface and documents soft tissue details but is applied only in selected patients (such as those with webs or stenoses) because of higher radiation exposure than in conventional techniques.

Except in an emergency, radiographic examination should be undertaken in children before the airways are inspected with use of general anesthesia. In most cases the airway can be seen from the nasal cavities above to the bifurcation of the trachea at the carina below, including clear details of the soft tissues of the larynx and pharynx.

As there is an enormous variation in the appearance of the normal in radiological studies, artifacts are commonly misinterpreted by the inexperienced. Radiographic study does not replace endoscopy in the assessment of the larynx and upper respiratory tract, but it does provide useful information prior to endoscopic examination. Interpretation must be made with the knowledge that the airways are dynamic structures, changing their appearance and diameter during different phases of respiration.

Tomography

In adults linear tomography and CT scan can be useful in malignant disease; in particular the anatomical details of a mass in the glottic, subglottic, or upper tracheal region can be identified to plan treatment and in advanced cases to judge the amount of airway obstruction to be expected during induction and maintenance of anesthesia.

CT scan of the neck shows extension of neoplastic disease into the pre-epiglottic space or outside the framework of the larynx, especially if the cartilages are ossified. Unsuspected or doubtful metastases in the lateral neck may be identified. Various cysts and soft tissue space infections and abscesses can be seen. Studies in the contrast phase are useful in vascular lesions. Tomography has been usefully applied to the larynx and neck in children in selected cases only, such as cystic hygroma, tumor, or pharyngeal space infection.

INSTRUMENTS AND EQUIPMENT

The first esophagoscopy was performed in 1868 by Kussmaul in Germany on a professional sword swallower. Thereafter Killian, also in Germany, and Chevalier Jackson in the United States developed endoscopes for bronchoscopy and laryngoscopy. Design modifications over the last 100 years have improved the instruments, but the major technological advances have been (1) image magnification using optical telescopes, (2) the operating microscope, and (3) flexible fiberoptics. The modern preference is for cold light fountains and flexible light-carrying cables to provide brilliant, cold light delivered to the endoscope as either proximal or distal illumination.

Illumination

Halogen Light Source. There are many light sources available; the most useful is a cold light fountain with two outlets. Bright illumination from a 250-watt halogen lamp has a color temperature of approximately 3,400K, and the light intensity is adjustable in increasing steps of brightness. There is a built-in second, spare lamp which can be switched on within seconds if the first lamp fails so that the examination will not be interrupted. Each of the two light outlets can be used simultaneously, for instance, for a laryngoscope and a bronchoscope or a laryngoscope and a telescope. This facility is essential for a patient with a partly obstructed airway; use of a laryngoscope may be necessary to ensure swift entry of a bronchoscope or an endotracheal tube for immediate ventilation and resuscitation.

Xenon Light Source. A xenon light source provides very bright illumination adjustable over a wide range and with a color temperature over 6,000K (approximately daylight brightness), so that daylight photographic film can be used for optimum clarity and color rendition. The xenon light fountain is preferred for television, videodocumentation, and cinephotography. A xenon light source is available that not only gives constant illumination for documentation but also provides pulsed automatically regulated, synchronized, reliable illumination for single-frame 35-mm photography.

Flash for Photography. There are several systems available for single-frame 35-mm photography with either electronic flash or high-intensity light. One such relatively inexpensive system consists of a small, sealed electronic flash tube that couples into the illumination system between the flexible fiberoptic cable and the telescope, but it is heavy and somewhat cumbersome. It has been replaced by a system that utilizes a more powerful flash generator and illumination system but is remote from the telescope and camera (Figure 1) and easier to use. The examining telescope receives continuous light through its fiberoptic light cable, and the synchronized flash pulse, generated in the computer-

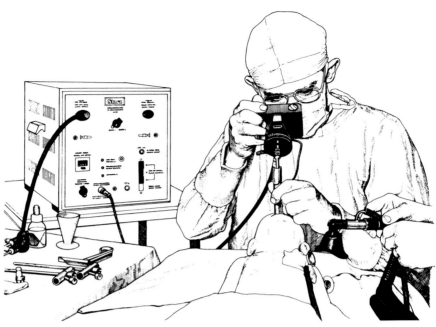

Figure 1. Photography of the larynx in an infant. The anesthetic face mask has been removed temporarily. The flash is transmitted along a fiberoptic cable from the light box, synchronized to the camera shutter by the connecting cord.

controlled flash unit, automatically delivers metered light through the same cable, the camera shutter being synchronized by a lightweight electrical cord.

Endoscopic Illumination. Originally makeshift lamps and then tiny electric bulbs in the distal end of the endoscopes provided illumination, but these have now been superseded. Proximal lighting is now delivered into the endoscope by a glass prism, a fiberoptic clip, or a single or double short fiberoptic rod. Distal lighting is brighter and is delivered through a thin round or oval rod incorporated into the wall of the laryngoscope or bronchoscope.

Flexible Endoscopes. The development of small fiberglass threads for transmission of light has been the most significant step in obtaining improved reliable "cold" illumination. When the glass fibers are sorted carefully into a coherent unit, an image can be transmitted even when the fiberglass bundle is in a curved or bent position; this has made flexible endoscopes feasible. The flexible nasopharyngolaryngoscopes for adults and children are a very valuable addition for the laryngologist, providing useful information when indirect mirror examination is not possible. The image is a collection of small dots and cannot equal the resolution and clarity obtained with mirror or rigid rod lens examination.

When the diameter of the flexible endoscope is decreased for pediatric application, the resolution of the image, although good, is a little less clear because there are fewer threads in the system. In flexible endoscopes less than 3 mm in diameter it is not possible to incorporate a control mechanism for the tip, a channel for suction, and a channel for instrumentation; therefore, although the small flexible instruments provide a good image, they do not have the capabilities of the adult instruments. Another disadvantage of the flexible endoscope in infants and small children with pre-existing airway obstruction is the inevitable added airway obstruction as the instrument is introduced.

Light-Carrying Cables. Fiberoptic light cables come in various diameters, lengths, and configurations, some being split into a Y-shape so that dual illumination can be obtained from a single light output although with some loss of brightness for each. Other cables have a reverse Y-shape so that extra-bright illumination can be obtained by having two sites of illumination directed into one cable.

Fluid light cables are available in various diameters and lengths but they cannot be made into a Y-shape. Fluid cables transmit light through a fluid medium, and the cable is less flexible than the standard fiberoptic cable. They offer the advantage of transmitting more light with a better color temperature and are recommended for documentation whether by still photography, cinephotography, or telerecording.

Rigid Telescopes

The coherent fiber bundles in the Hopkins rigid rod lens optical telescope system give superb resolution and contrast, natural color reproduction, a wide viewing angle, and bright light transmission even in a small-diameter instrument. The depth of the field for viewing or for photography is excellent. The detailed, magnified image allows a more extensive and complete examination of the laryngopharynx than is possible using a laryngoscope with the naked eye. A wide range of Hopkins rod lens telescopes is available, with diameters that vary from 2.7 to 10 mm, for use in various endoscopic instruments. The length is chosen according to the intended use, for example, a short telescope for examination of the nasal cavities or a very long telescope for esophagoscopy and bronchoscopy in adults. The standard angle of viewing is 0° and a wide viewing field can be provided. In others the angle of viewing is 30°, 50°, 70°, 90°, or 120° according to requirements, each having a wide field of view and excellent depth of focus.

Many ingenious instruments have been designed and put to practical use by incorporating slim telescopes for precise manipulations within body cavities, such as optical bronchoscopic forceps for grasping foreign bodies.

The technique of endoscopy to be described uses telescopes constantly, not only in the larynx but also in the tracheobronchial tree, esophagus, and nasal cavities. In the larynx, telescopes with a view angle of 0° or 30° provide superb clarity for evaluation. The dynamic changes of the tracheobronchial tree, especially in children, can be studied during spontaneous respiration under general anesthesia by using a slim telescope inserted through a laryngoscope into the trachea. In this way there is no distortion or distention of the trachea such as might occur using a rigid, open-tube bronchoscope or a wide-diameter flexible bronchoscope. Weak, collapsed, compressed, or stenosed areas can be identified using a telescope alone as a tracheoscope.

Laryngoscopes

There are many endoscopes available for examination of the upper respiratory tract, with a wide variety for the larynx. The laryngoscope is a fundamental tool for the laryngologist.

The laryngoscope is basically an open tube with illumination at either the proximal or the distal end of the instrument. Besides the general-purpose laryngoscopes for routine examination, there are special purpose laryngoscopes and microlaryngoscopes. Many of these have features providing an improved view of the vocal cords and the subglottic area. Some laryngoscopes have complicated mechanisms and may be difficult to use. Instruments with a straightforward design are advocated for diagnostic examination, biopsy, laser surgery, and other endoscopic manipulations.

ADULTS

The laryngoscopes favored for use in adults are:

1. *The Kleinsasser, Jako, Dedo, or Nagashima operating laryngoscopes* of various sizes are all-purpose instruments and are standard in many laryngology units. They are designed to expose and allow examination of the glottic opening. There are, of course, many other laryngoscopes available; each has its advantages and disadvantages, and personal preference will indicate the choice. The requirements include a wide proximal end for binocular vision; easy entry of instruments; safe use of the laser; a distal end of suitable size to expose the area of the larynx being investigated or operated upon without trauma; and adaptation for anesthesia, whether it be insufflation anesthesia, jet anesthesia, or anesthesia using an endotracheal tube.

2. *The Lindholm operating laryngoscope* (Figure 2). The unique design of this instrument is helpful in pharyngeal and laryngeal examination and surgical treatment of both adults and children, providing a panoramic view of the laryngopharynx, including excellent views of

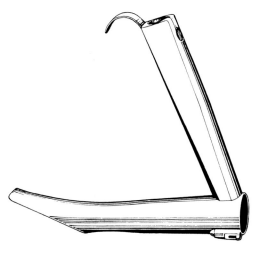

Figure 2. Lindholm operating laryngoscope for adults and children.

the vocal cords, endolarynx, epiglottis, aryepiglottic folds, arytenoids, piriform fossae, and postcricoid region. The beak of the laryngoscope is placed at the base of the tongue in the valleculae in front of the epiglottis, and the ''hourglass'' shape permits an overall view of the larynx and pharynx.

It is an excellent instrument for endolaryngeal surgery such as arytenoidectomy, removal of supraglottic tumors and cysts, laser excision of supraglottic papillomas, and examination and biopsy of lesions of the piriform fossae or of the supraglottic or posterior pharyngeal wall.

3. *The Benjamin slimline binocular operating microlaryngoscope* (Figure 3) has a distal shape and size similar to that of the standard Holinger adult anterior commissure laryngoscope, but the proximal opening of this new laryngoscope is oval with side-to-side dimensions sufficiently wide for binocular viewing using the operating microscope. The dimensions are compatible with binocular stereoscopic observation and use of the carbon dioxide laser, and yet the instrument is narrow enough to allow examination of the larynx when other, larger instruments have failed. It is an essential additional instrument for use in adult patients in whom the larynx is difficult or impossible to visualize with standard microlaryngoscopes.

4. *The Holinger anterior commissure laryngoscope, adult size* has distal fiberoptic illumination and is the best available instrument for examination of the larynx in difficult situations. However, it allows only monocular viewing and cannot be used satisfactorily with the operating microscope or with the laser. The anterior commissure, the subglottic region, and the posterior glottis can be examined with this instrument.

Although each operating microlaryngoscope is supplied with its own separate fiberoptic light carrier made to fit each particular laryngoscope, the Benjamin-Havas universal fiberoptic lighting clip (Figure 3) can be used to provide bright lighting. This clip attaches instantly to the right-hand side of any laryngoscope and is convenient for changing from one laryngoscope to another. Once a suitable-sized laryngoscope for microlaryngoscopy has been positioned, it is held by a self-retaining

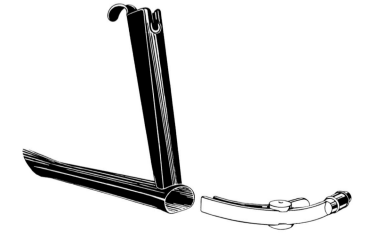

Figure 3. Benjamin slimline binocular operating microlaryngoscope for adults. The Benjamin-Havas universal fiberoptic lighting clip is also shown.

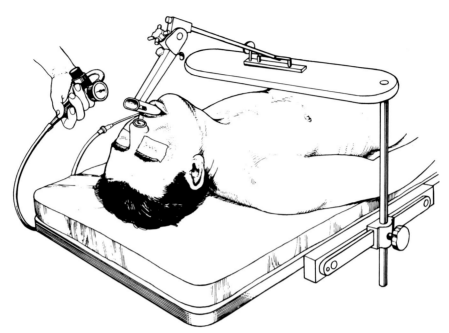

Figure 4. The distal cross-plate of the self-retaining laryngoscope holder rests squarely on the Mustard table, which itself is clear of the chest and firmly fixed to the operating table. Note the jetting tube for anesthesia.

laryngoscope holder (Figure 4), which is adjusted into place so that two hands are available for endolaryngeal manipulation.

The adjustable self-retaining microlaryngoscope holder rests firmly on a Mustard table (Figure 4), which itself is clamped firmly to the side of the operating table. The whole assembly moves as a unit when the operating table is raised, lowered, or tilted. The base plate of the self-retaining holder should not lie on the patient's chest, where it could restrict respiration and significantly affect conditions of anesthesia.

CHILDREN

There are a number of different laryngoscopes for pediatric use:

1. *Standard laryngoscopes* for general use. These diagnostic instruments are open-sided for introduction of a bronchoscope or an endotracheal tube. The Storz slotted pediatric laryngoscopes (Figure 5) of 8.0, 9.5, 11.0, and 13.5 cm length have lighting by a proximal prism. The Jackson pediatric laryngoscopes with a slide and distal lighting by a fiberoptic rod are a suitable alternative.
2. The *Holinger pediatric anterior commissure* laryngoscope (Figure 6), which is 11 cm long, is essential for a larynx that is difficult to expose or examine. A modified version is available that is slotted to allow intubation.
3. The *Tucker-Benjamin slotted neonatal laryngoscope and subglottiscope* is only 9.0 cm long and is for use in premature and newborn babies. This slim laryngoscope is used to examine the anterior and the posterior commissure and the interarytenoid regions. Deliberately

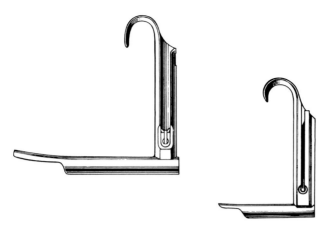

Figure 5. The largest (13.5 cm) and the smallest (8.0 cm) standard Storz slotted pediatric laryngoscopes.

separating the vocal folds allows more satisfactory visualization of the subglottic region than is obtained with other instruments.

4. *The Lindholm operating microlaryngoscope* (Figure 2) described previously was designed for adults; despite its size, it gives superb exposure, without trauma, in infants from 6 to 9 months of age.

5. *Operating microlaryngoscopes.* For microlaryngoscopy and microlaryngeal surgery, the suspension technique is used. Both the Lindholm operating laryngoscope and the large and small *Benjamin pediatric operating microlaryngoscopes* (Figure 7) provide clear binocular vision.

6. *The Healy subglottiscope* is for microsurgery or laser surgery in the subglottic region in infants. Its narrow distal barrel separates and protects the vocal cords during treatment of subglottic or upper tracheal pathology such as papilloma or hemangioma.

Microsurgical Instruments

Shorter microlaryngoscopy instruments allow more precise use with increased manual stability and diminished tremor. These new instruments have reinforced shafts that are 18 cm long, compared with the conventional 25 cm, and are suitable for both adult and pediatric use. They have a firm action and a positive feel, and the shorter shaft is more easily introduced into a laryngoscope when the laser attachment is on the microscope.

There are straight-ahead, right, left, and up-cupped forceps in a

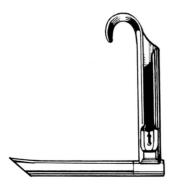

Figure 6. The Holinger pediatric anterior commissure laryngoscope.

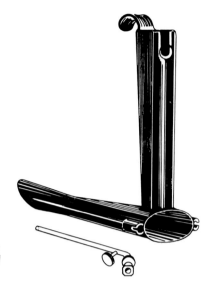

Figure 7. The Benjamin pediatric operating microlaryngoscope. Anesthetic gases are delivered down the side channel through the metal cannula.

variety of cup sizes and shapes; various grasping forceps; straight-ahead, up-tilted, curved right and left scissors; various specialized grasping and foreign body forceps; needle-holding forceps; suckers with beaded, atraumatic tips; and diathermy with suction.

For injection of Teflon or Gelfoam paste into the larynx there is a high-pressure syringe "gun" with click stops and clear markings to indicate the volume injected. A reinforced high-pressure injection cannula with a 19-FG, 20-cm needle beveled at 45° is used.

The Carbon Dioxide Laser

Clinical application of the carbon dioxide laser in surgery of the upper airways enables a fine laser beam to be accurately directed to any part of the field seen with the operating microscope. A helium-neon aiming beam indicates the treatment site, and a micromanipulator mounted on the microscope allows each laser exposure to be precisely placed.

The microsurgical laser, used in both adult and pediatric laryngology, allows precise vaporization of various lesions with constant visual control of the beam, virtual absence of bleeding, little reactive edema, and minimal postoperative pain. The carbon dioxide laser is particularly suitable for vaporization of laryngeal papilloma; there is little or no bleeding, so treatment at more than one site can be performed at each operation, whereas when forceps or scissors are used, bleeding tends to obscure the operative site. During the final stage of papilloma removal it is not uncommon to require small, cupped forceps angled left, right, or upward to remove residual papillomas from areas such as the laryngeal ventricle or the anterior commissure. Alternatively, in these difficult anatomical sites the laser beam can be reflected onto the lesion by using a small metal mirror.

The laser is also suitable for treatment of some congenital and acquired webs and stenoses, hemangiomas, lymphangiomas, epithelial dysplasias, easily accessible early malignancies in adults, granulomas, and laryngeal amyloid, and for arytenoidectomy and removal of other selected tumors.

Mini Microlaryngeal Surgery

A microspot micromanipulator developed by Shapshay and others has improved precise application of the carbon dioxide laser in the larynx. The small spot is about one-third the diameter produced by conventional instruments. During microlaryngeal procedures with this spot the increased power density minimizes surrounding tissue trauma and allows laser power reduction to 1 watt or less for incisions approximately 300 μm in width. An additional feature of this micromanipulator system is a "power defocus" mechanism for hemostasis and less precise tissue ablation. A small button on the end of the joystick can be depressed to activate an optical system that shortens the focal length of the lens system to one of five predetermined positions. This new system features a fiberoptic aiming light, thus avoiding the conventional helium-neon laser coincident aiming beam, which can create a disturbing glare effect on tissue.

Microspot laser surgery using microflap and microwelding techniques are possible when used in conjunction with the newly designed Shapshay/Healy mini microlaryngoscopy instruments. This set of smaller, 1- to 2-mm instruments has 20-cm triple-reinforced shafts, and the forceps, scissors, and suction tubes are designed for precision techniques such as:

- Removal of benign lesions with less trauma
- Endoscopic flap techniques
- Tissue microwelding
- Pediatric laryngeal surgery in newborns and infants

The technique is recommended for vocal cord polyps, Reinke's edema, dysplasias, selected benign and malignant tumors, and glottic and subglottic stenoses. In selected stenoses a mucosal flap is elevated, the stenotic tissue is excised, and the flap is reapplied using the microspot laser welding technique.

The final place of mini microlaryngeal surgery will not be known for some time yet.

Teaching and Documentation

USING TELESCOPES

An assistant or a student may observe the exact image seen through the telescope by the endoscopist by using a teaching attachment. The Hopkins rod lens system permits splitting of the reflected image while maintaining adequate brightness of the image for each of two simultaneous observers.

The Wittmoser multiarticulated optical arm (Figure 8) has four joints, and although the most expensive, it is undoubtedly the best optical observer and documentation arm. The dual beam splitter can be switched from 50%–50% for the examiner and observer to 10%–90%

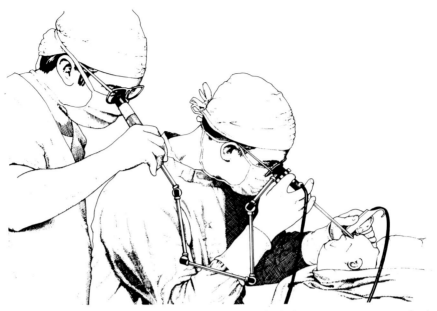

Figure 8. An assistant using the Wittmoser optical observer arm sees exactly the same view as the surgeon.

for documentation using a 35-mm still camera, a cinecamera, or a television camera. There is natural color reproduction, superb image quality, complete safety for the patient, and no interference to the endoscopist.

USING THE MICROSCOPE

During microlaryngoscopy or microlaryngeal surgery a beam splitter allows observation by an assistant (Figure 9), 35-mm still photogra-

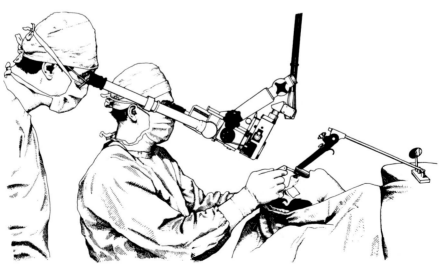

Figure 9. An assistant using the observer arm mounted on the beam splitter of the microscope.

phy, cinephotography, or endoscopic video monitoring and recording. Observation is confined to the larynx; there is not the flexibility of endoscopic visualization that is available with telescopes that can be passed into the nasal cavities, paranasal sinuses, postnasal space, pharynx, larynx, trachea, bronchi, and esophagus.

VIDEO MONITORING

Using a small television camera with high resolution and low light sensitivity on the telescope or the microscope, the anesthesiologist, nursing staff, and assistants can observe the endoscopic procedure. The anesthesiologist is able to monitor the airway and observe the conditions of anesthesia, the instrument nurse can anticipate the progress of the procedure, and the operating room staff feel more involvement in the operations. Routine endoscopic observation, teaching, and documentation are now an everyday routine, with a suitable video recorder used for permanent documentation.

PHOTOGRAPHY

Many methods of laryngeal photography have been used successfully for both black and white and color reproductions using 35-mm single-frame photography. The most consistently reliable and versatile system producing good quality laryngeal photographs utilizes a 35-mm single-frame reflex camera with the Hopkins' telescopes and a synchro-

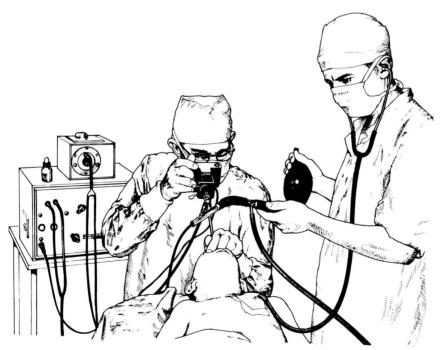

Figure 10. Photography in the tracheobronchial tree using a telescope passed through a ventilating bronchoscope.

nized, automatic exposure electronic flash generator (Figure 10). Consistently reproducible photographic documentation under both good and adverse conditions is a practical reality using standard film and processing, and the system maintains complete safety for the patient, even in small infants or where there is partial or severe airway obstruction.

For video display and cinephotography a xenon light source provides continuous extra-bright illumination, which is especially necessary when the small 2.7-mm diameter telescopes are used. The video recorder (the 0.75-inch U-matic system is preferred) should provide a still-frame feature, forward and backward search scanning, playback, and programmed access to stored information.

ANESTHESIA FOR LARYNGOSCOPY

It is possible to accomplish direct laryngoscopy without general anesthesia by using topical and nerve block local anesthesia. Local anesthesia properly applied to the mucosa of the oral cavity, pharynx, and larynx allows the endoscopist to perform open tube diagnostic examination and biopsy with little discomfort for some cooperative patients. However, general anesthesia is preferable, especially for extended examinations, for surgical and microsurgical procedures, and for patients who are unsuitable for local anesthesia because of anatomical variants or undue anxiety. General anesthesia gives the best conditions for the surgeon and the least discomfort for the patient.

In modern practice general anesthesia is now used almost universally for direct laryngoscopy, microlaryngoscopy, and microlaryngeal operations, including laser surgery. Examination of the tracheobronchial tree and the esophagus can be performed with modifications of the technique used for laryngoscopy. The chosen anesthetic technique must ensure safety and yet minimally impede visual and surgical access. Some techniques require the use of an endotracheal tube, and others do not; in some cases a modified endotracheal tube or a jetting system can be used.

For adult laryngoscopy a relaxant technique with controlled ventilation is preferred. For pediatric endoscopy spontaneous respiration with inhalational anesthesia is preferred. In all patients general anesthesia is supplemented by the use of a measured amount of topical lidocaine sprayed on the larynx and upper trachea.

With advances in endoscopy, especially the advent of microlaryngoscopy, many ingenious methods of general anesthesia have evolved. The choice of technique will depend on the anesthetic agents available, the method of ventilation to be used, the state of the patient's general health, the actual procedure to be performed, and the preference of the surgeon. For example there are different requirements for an infant in the investigation of stridor, for laryngoscopy and biopsy of a malignant tumor causing partial airway obstruction in an adult, for panendoscopy for a suspected but unproven upper respiratory tract tumor, for microlaryngoscopy and surgical removal of a vocal nodule, and for carbon dioxide laser surgery with destruction or excision of diseased tissue. Each patient and each procedure presents a different problem. The techniques of anesthesia used must not only encompass the range of laryngeal, endoscopic, and microsurgical procedures but must be suitable for patients of all ages—premature babies, infants, children, adults, and geriatric patients.

The ideal requirements for safe anesthesia include:

- Simple, rapid induction and prompt, comfortable recovery
- Control of secretions and blood
- An immobile, unobstructed larynx during operative procedures
- No time restriction for surgical procedures or for documentation

- Conditions that allow observation of the dynamics of the larynx, usually at the end of the procedure
- Minimal chance of aspiration
- Safe use of the laser

These ideals must be compatible with maximum safety and minimum patient discomfort.

Many demanding problems confront the endoscopist and the anesthesiologist, sometimes quite unexpectedly, so that mutual confidence, understanding, and teamwork are essential to safely share access to a limited airway. All anesthetic techniques for laryngoscopy have their own disadvantages and complications. The potential problems for a particular procedure must be discussed by the anesthesiologist and the surgeon so that each is forewarned of the possible difficulties and can plan means of overcoming them.

Anesthesia Techniques for Adults

General anesthetic techniques without intubation are difficult to apply in adults. Apneic techniques as well as methods making use of a cuirass respirator or a volatile inhalational agent such as ether have been tried, but each has been discarded. The techniques of general anesthesia for microlaryngeal surgery that are in use today generally involve endotracheal intubation, use of a catheter for insufflation of anesthetic gases, or specially designed tubes for high-pressure jetting either proximally into the lumen of the laryngoscope or distally with the tube in the lumen of the trachea.

The endotracheal tube may be cuffed or uncuffed, and of small or large diameter. For laser surgery the tube can be protected by a "laser-proof" coating or by wrapping it with aluminum foil strips, or a metal tube can be used. Complete surgical exposure of the larynx and subglottic area cannot be obtained using a standard endotracheal tube, as the tube obscures the posterior part of the larynx and the subglottic region. In selected cases a small-diameter "microlaryngoscopy" tube may be preferred by the anesthesiologist and be acceptable to the endoscopist, particularly when the disease is known to be supraglottic or in the anterior part of the larynx.

ANESTHESIA FOR LASER USE

The problem of laser ignition and combustion of a tube during microlaryngeal laser surgery has not been satisfactorily solved. Most metal tubes are thick-walled, cumbersome, and to some degree traumatic to the larynx and trachea, and do not provide optimal exposure. The new Laser-Flex cuffed tracheal tube is an improvement. It is made of stainless steel with a soft plastic distal segment and two cuffs that can be inflated with isotonic saline. Tubes wrapped in aluminum foil or coated with a "laser-proof" coating give some protection. However, these cannot be given an unqualified recommendation, because the cuff and the unprotected parts of the tube may be at risk since the foil may not adhere to the tube and the coating does not give dependable protection. Indiscriminate or careless laser surgery with a metal tube or an aluminum-wrapped tube has caused superheating with consequent thermal burn. The only universally satisfactory method would be not to use an anesthetic tube; although this ideal is readily available in infants and children, the technique cannot be satisfactorily applied to adults. Helium gas has a high thermal diffusivity, and use of a 40% oxygen and 60% helium gas mixture will delay the start of a potential laser-induced fire in a plastic anesthetic tube.

JET ANESTHESIA

There are many methods that utilize the Venturi jet technique with regular bursts of high-pressure oxygen or oxygen–nitrous oxide mixture. With jet ventilation, according to preference, the tip of the jetting device can be in the proximal opening of the laryngoscope, in the subglottic region, or in the mid-trachea. The most important complication of jet ventilation is barotrauma with subsequent pneumomediastinum or pneumothorax.

General anesthesia with a muscle relaxant achieves nearly ideal conditions when a peroral translaryngeal endotracheal catheter of very small diameter is used to maintain adequate gas exchange. We use the Benjamin jet (Benjet) anesthesia tube, a specially designed, very small diameter jet tube for almost all adults (Figure 11). The outside diameter of the tube is 2.8 mm. It is easy to introduce and remove, cannot be kinked or obstructed, and is unobtrusive in the larynx. The surgeon has an excellent view of the surgical field, as the tube normally lies inconspicuously in the posterior commissure (Figure 12A). The tube can be displaced by the laryngoscope to the anterior commissure for work in the posterior part of the glottis.

When laser surgery is being used the tube can be protected by a moist cottonoid, but its position in the subglottic region and trachea must be constantly noted so that it will not be struck by the laser beam.

Correct placement is assessed visually, a mark on the tube at the glottic level acting as a guide so that the distal end of the tube is maintained in the mid-trachea. Even distribution of gases is assured because the distal tip is centrally located in the trachea (Figure 13), stabilized by the four soft plastic petals so that it cannot impinge on the tracheal mucosa to cause a traumatic laceration. The potential complication of a jet blast causing rupture of the airway can be avoided.

Jet ventilation *is not commenced* until a laryngoscope is placed to view the glottic opening and ensure expiration. Ventilation of both lungs

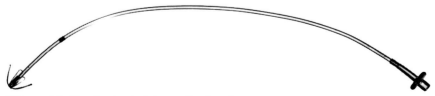

Figure 11. The Benjamin jet anesthesia tube.

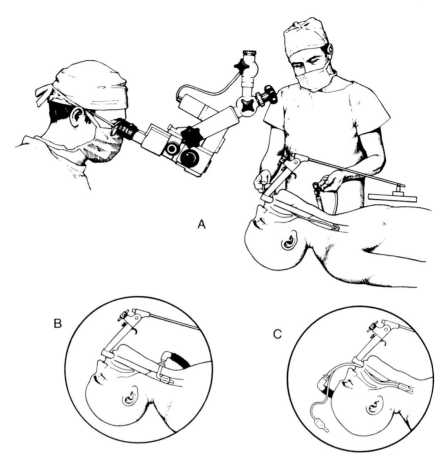

Figure 12. Anesthesia techniques for laryngoscopy and microlaryngoscopy in adults. *A*, Jet ventilation using the Benjamin jet tube positioned in the mid-trachea. *B*, Tracheotomy tube. *C*, Small-diameter cuffed microlaryngoscopy endotracheal tube.

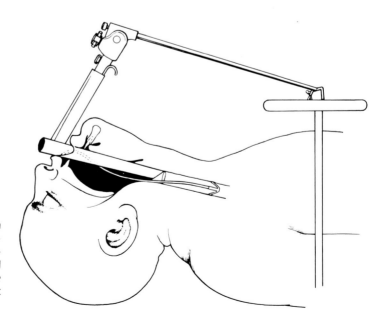

Figure 13. The jet ventilation tube (2.8 mm outside diameter) lies in the posterior laryngeal commissure and the distal tip is centrally located in the trachea, stabilized by four soft plastic petals.

is immediately checked by using auscultation and movement of the chest as the guides to adequate ventilation before the tube is fixed to the face by strapping (Figure 14). Special care must be taken in obese patients and those with poor lung and chest wall compliance. One hundred percent oxygen is used for jet ventilation. A 40% oxygen and 60% helium mixture is used during laser surgery.

Maintenance of anesthesia is by continuous intravenous infusion of a short-acting barbiturate such as methohexital or the newer agent propofol together with either a continuous infusion of succinylcholine or use of a short-acting nondepolarizing relaxant.

The expiratory phase must be unimpaired at all times. A soft plastic nasopharyngeal tube placed in one nasal cavity (Figure 14) maintains the pharyngeal and nasal airway. Use of the Benjet tube is contraindicated in the presence of significant laryngeal obstruction such as an obstructing carcinoma or a large mass of papilloma.

We find the Benjet tube especially useful for laser surgery in the larynx. Although potentially flammable after laser ignition in a low-flow oxygen environment, a tube of such small diameter can be easily displaced into the anterior or posterior part of the larynx so that, with vigilance by the operator, the laser beam may be used at a safe distance from it.

Jet ventilation with a short-acting relaxant makes injection of a vocal cord with Teflon or Gelfoam paste with the patient under general anesthesia an acceptable and accurate technique. There is no endotracheal tube to obstruct or distort accurate placement of the paste. Cessation of the relaxant allows vocal cord movement to return so that adequacy of placement of the paste can be judged precisely. All jetting must be stopped before the glottis closes and obstructs expiration as spontaneous respiration resumes.

We have used this jet technique for laryngoscopy, microlaryngoscopy, and microlaryngeal surgery for over 10 years without complication. No tube has been ignited and there have been no barotrauma

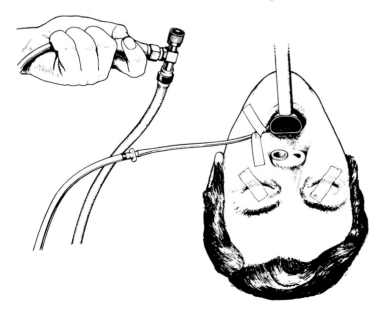

Figure 14. Detailed view of the jet tube in use, fixed to the face by strapping. The proximal end is securely attached to the jet injector equipment. Note the nasopharyngeal airway.

complications. However, anesthetic techniques that use high-pressure jet ventilation should be employed only by an experienced anesthesiologist and surgeon who are able to recognize the potential complications.

RELAXANT TECHNIQUE WITH A MICROLARYNGOSCOPY TUBE

The most commonly used tube is a cuffed polyvinylchloride microlaryngoscopy endotracheal tube (Figure 12C). Microlaryngoscopy tubes are manufactured with inside diameters of 4.0, 5.0, and 6.0 mm. A tube is chosen with as small a diameter as will allow satisfactory ventilation even though there is some increased airway resistance. The tube is 30 cm long, the extra length being helpful to lead it from the side of the mouth away from the laryngoscope. Despite its smaller diameter, a cuffed microlaryngoscopy tube allows predictable ventilation and may be preferred where there is pre-existing upper airway obstruction, where intubation is desired to secure safe ventilation, in "poor risk" patients with pre-existing respiratory or cardiovascular disease, and when an anesthesiologist is working with an endoscopist whose technique is not known to him, perhaps in unfamiliar surroundings.

Anesthesia in patients who have a tracheotomy is uncomplicated and requires no special consideration (Figure 12B).

No matter which anesthesic technique is being used, a measured amount of topical anesthetic solution, up to 5 mg per kg of lidocaine, is applied to the laryngeal mucous membrane using a metered aerosol spray that delivers 10 mg of lidocaine per spray.

Anesthesia Techniques for Infants and Children

Diagnostic endoscopy in either infants or children is very seldom carried out without general anesthesia. It may occasionally be safer to carry out "cold" orotracheal intubation without any form of anesthesia in a sick neonate or, for example, a baby with a difficult airway problem such as can occur in the Pierre Robin syndrome.

General anesthesia without an endotracheal tube provides ideal conditions for endoscopic examination. When it becomes necessary to use a tube (Figure 15C), visualization of the anterior part of the larynx is adequate but even a small-diameter tube obstructs the view of the posterior part of the larynx and the subglottic region and precludes accurate assessment of laryngeal movement. In cases with severe obstruction, for example large papillomas or a subglottic hemangioma, intubation may be necessary initially to secure the airway, stabilize anesthesia, and allow thorough assessment of the pathological condition before planning further management.

General anesthesia without an endotracheal tube is therefore the method of choice for endoscopy of the larynx and tracheobronchial tree. An inhalational technique (Figure 16) relying entirely on spontaneous respiration utilizing oxygen, nitrous oxide, halothane, and topical anesthesia does not require an endotracheal tube. Another method relies on

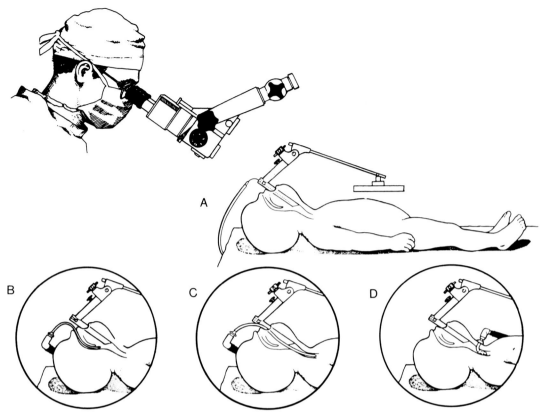

Figure 15. Anesthesia techniques for laryngoscopy and microlaryngoscopy in infants and children, with anesthetic gases delivered (A) through a metal cannula in the side of the laryngoscope, (B) through a nasopharyngeal tube, (C) through a narrow endotracheal tube, and (D) through a tracheotomy tube.

insufflation into the oropharynx via a tube passed through one nasal cavity (Figure 15B), but it may be difficult to maintain a steady level of anesthesia. Some anesthesiologists prefer to add methoxyflurane to the gaseous mixture, regarding it as a supplement to provide additional analgesia that "smoothes out" the procedure. In the case of an ill child, oxygen with halothane would be used, omitting the nitrous oxide.

This spontaneous-respiration technique gives unrestricted access to all parts of the airway, and there is the benefit of unhurried assessment of vocal cord movements and laryngeal dynamics. Tracheobronchoscopy can be performed using a ventilating bronchoscope with gaseous exchange taking place to maintain anesthesia through the open tube bronchoscope while it is in the tracheobronchial tree. When examination of the nasopharynx or the esophagus is required, a peroral endotracheal tube is used to secure the airway. With this inhalational method no satisfactory technique for scavenging anesthetic gases is currently available.

Anesthesia through a tracheotomy tube (Figure 15D) gives ideal conditions for laryngoscopy.

For premedication atropine alone is used for babies and for most older children. In selected older children the combination of either meperidine and atropine or papaverine hydrochloride and scopolamine

ANESTHESIA FOR ENDOSCOPY

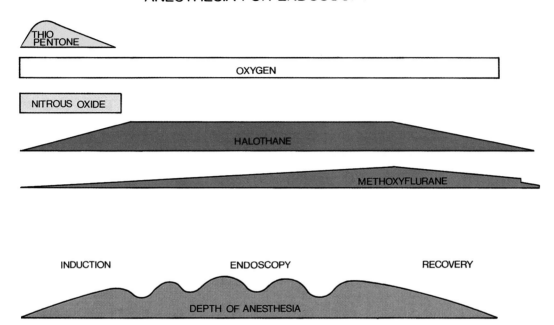

Figure 16. Spontaneous-respiration general anesthesia for pediatric endoscopy. Induction may be accomplished either with an intravenous agent or by inhalation with a face mask using nitrous oxide, oxygen, and halothane, often supplemented by methoxyflurane. The depth of anesthesia varies as local anesthetic solution is applied and as the various endoscopes are introduced.

is used, with the precaution that a narcotic is not administered in the presence of respiratory obstruction. If atropine has not been given by intramuscular injection, it is given intravenously at or soon after induction; atropine affords protection against bradycardia and minimizes secretions in the respiratory tract.

Induction may be accomplished with intravenous thiopental or similar agent or by inhalation with a face mask, but in either case a venipuncture is always performed to secure an intravenous route. A muscle relaxant is drawn up to be given if required, for example, for a persistent or uncontrolled laryngeal spasm or for removal of a difficult foreign body.

Topical anesthesia up to a maximum of 5 mg per kg of lidocaine is used as a 4% solution in children, but in infants it is usually diluted with saline to a 1% or 2% concentration to give sufficient volume that can be handled conveniently. Using a syringe and a Cass needle (Figure 27) it is sprayed onto the epiglottis, larynx, and upper trachea to minimize unwanted reflex activity. This combination of general and local anesthesia is most important, as it virtually abolishes laryngeal spasm during and after endoscopy.

Anesthetic gases are stopped altogether at the end of the diagnostic procedure, and oxygen alone is administered by a small-diameter tube (Figure 15B) passed through the nose into the pharynx. Direct laryngoscopy is continued to allow observation of the dynamics of laryngeal movement, for example, in patients with laryngomalacia or vocal cord paralysis.

The standard technique for microlaryngoscopy delivers anesthetic gases through a wide-bore cannula (Figure 15A) inserted into a side channel in the laryngoscope (Figure 7) for insufflation close to the glottic opening, thus maintaining a high concentration. To minimize contamination of the trachea with blood, mucus, or foreign tissue, careful suctioning is performed from time to time. Absolutely clear access to the larynx is obtained without the obstruction of a tube, making this method especially useful for laser surgery.

Anesthesia is easily maintained at an adequate depth by insufflation and spontaneous respiration in children up to 12 years of age, but over this age the techniques applying to adults usually become necessary.

TECHNIQUE OF ENDOSCOPY

There have been many advances since laryngoscopy was first developed over 100 years ago. Not only have there been major improvements in the design of the endoscopes themselves, but general anesthesia is widely available, laryngeal microsurgery has evolved, flexible fiberoptic light-carrying leads have been developed, flexible endoscopes have been universally accepted, and the applications of rigid fiberoptic telescopes have been expanded.

The technique of laryngoscopy will be described first for adults, and then similar methods will be described for infants and children. Additional descriptions for tracheobronchoscopy, esophagoscopy, and examination of the nasal cavities and nasopharynx will also be given.

Technique in Adults

The task of performing a great number of bronchoscopic examinations in adults has passed from the otolaryngologists to our colleagues in thoracic medicine and surgery who have the necessary expertise and training in flexible fiberoptic instruments and who undertake the continuing care of the patient. The otolaryngologist remains the clinician trained and experienced in direct laryngoscopy, endoscopic microlaryngeal surgery, and carbon dioxide laser treatment in the upper airways.

In adults with malignant disease in the laryngopharynx, in addition to laryngoscopy, examination and palpation of the oral cavity, base of tongue, and tonsils together with complete tracheobronchoscopy and esophagoscopy are necessary to detect a possible second primary lesion.

General anesthesia for adults utilizes a muscle relaxant to paralyze the patient. A modified endotracheal tube such as a cuffed microlaryngoscopy tube, a tube for jet ventilation, or a tube modified for safe use with the laser is positioned. The design and pattern of the laryngoscope must be compatible with the technique of anesthesia and at the same time permit optimum exposure of the laryngeal structures.

There are three stages in laryngoscopy: direct laryngoscopy, laryngoscopy with telescopes, and microlaryngoscopy.

FIRST STAGE—DIRECT LARYNGOSCOPY

Direct laryngoscopy with the naked eye viewing through an open tube laryngoscope is the initial diagnostic procedure for examination of the larynx and pharynx. The *Lindholm microlaryngoscope* (Figure 2) is recommended as a suitable laryngoscope for a panoramic view of the laryngopharynx in most patients. The distal tip of the laryngoscope is placed in front of the epiglottis to display an overall view not only of the vocal cords and the endolarynx but also of the epiglottis, aryepiglottic folds, arytenoids, piriform fossae, and part of the postcricoid region. These areas can be clearly and easily inspected at direct laryngoscopy,

33

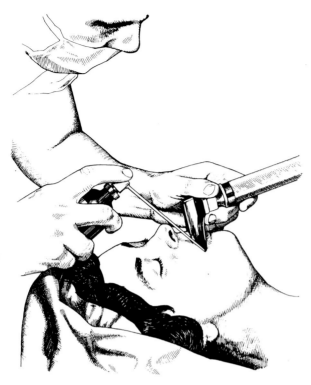

Figure 17. Application of a topical anesthetic solution using a metered aerosol spray.

with telescopes or the operating microscope, using the Lindholm laryngoscope. However, there are many different examining and operating laryngoscopes available according to personal preference, and each has its advantages and disadvantages.

Special-purpose laryngoscopes are required in adults when the larynx is difficult or impossible to visualize with standard instruments. The adult *Holinger anterior commissure laryngoscope* gives access in patients in whom the anatomy of the teeth, pharynx, and neck makes laryngoscope difficult. It is not applicable to microlaryngoscopy, as its narrow barrel allows only monocular vision, but image magnification with telescopes readily gives more information. The *Benjamin slimline binocular operating microlaryngoscope* (Figure 3) is similar to the Holinger but has a wider proximal end whose side-to-side dimensions are sufficient for binocular viewing using the microscope.

After anesthesia has been induced, a measured amount of topical anesthetic solution is applied (Figure 17) using a metered aerosol spray. The endotracheal tube or jetting tube is then positioned and the patient is ready for diagnostic examination.

The teeth are protected, and the laryngoscope, illuminated by the lighting clip (Figure 18), is passed through the right side of the mouth. As the base of the tongue is lifted forward, the epiglottis and the larynx can be seen. A "lever" action against the teeth is not used; the laryngoscope should be lifted.

The pharynx and larynx are then systematically evaluated. External pressure on the neck and gentle repositioning of the laryngoscope allows various areas of the larynx to be more prominently displayed. One or other vocal fold can be "rolled" to see the undersurface, and the false cord can be partly pushed aside to see more of the upper surface of the

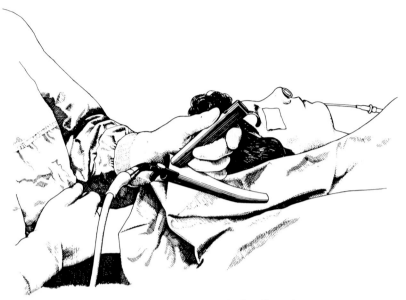

Figure 18. A Lindholm laryngoscope ready for direct laryngoscopy.

vocal fold. Mobility of the arytenoids at the cricoarytenoid joints is assessed using a blunt instrument to move the arytenoid (see page 56).

SECOND STAGE—LARYNGOSCOPY WITH TELESCOPES

The second stage of laryngoscopy requires image magnification using rigid telescopes to provide a more precise and comprehensive evaluation. All areas are evaluated using Hopkins rigid rod lens telescopes passed through either a hand-held laryngoscope or a laryngoscope suspended in position by a laryngoscope holder (Figure 19). Using the Lindholm laryngoscope, for example, the distribution of papillomas

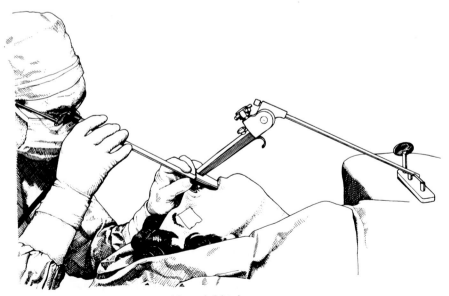

Figure 19. Laryngoscopy with a rigid telescope.

in the laryngopharynx or the site and size of a tumor or cyst can be delineated.

A 0° straight-ahead rigid telescope gives a close-up, wide-angled magnified image. Using a 30° or a 50° angled telescope the laryngeal ventricles, the anterior and posterior commisure, and the anterior subglottic region can be inspected in detail. A Wittmoser articulated optical arm reveals the exact view of the endoscopist to an assistant (Figure 20). Telescopes allow a more extensive and complete examination of the pharynx, larynx, and trachea than is possible with microlaryngoscopy; once a microlaryngoscope is fixed in position, using the microscope only, visualization of the laryngeal structures other than the glottis is limited. The ventricles and subglottic region cannot be fully inspected.

Telescopes provide precise and comprehensive information about the airway from the pharynx down to the carina. A 35-mm camera can be readily attached to the proximal end of the telescope (Figure 21) for single-frame photography.

This survey of the oropharynx, larynx, and subglottic region with rigid telescopes is a routine part of diagnostic laryngoscopy. In some cases the findings indicate the need to proceed to microlaryngoscopy and laryngeal surgery.

THIRD STAGE—MICROLARYNGOSCOPY

Microlaryngoscopy offers variable magnification, brilliant illumination, binocular vision, precise surgical manipulation, and freedom to use both hands for other procedures.

For illumination while positioning a microlaryngoscope, the Benjamin-Havas clip is used. It attaches to the right-hand side of the laryngoscope (Figure 3 and Figure 18) and readily provides light for any

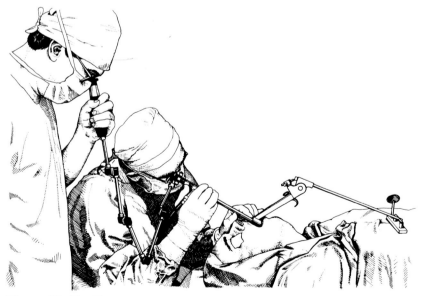

Figure 20. The Wittmoser optical teaching arm gives an observer the same clear view as that of the surgeon.

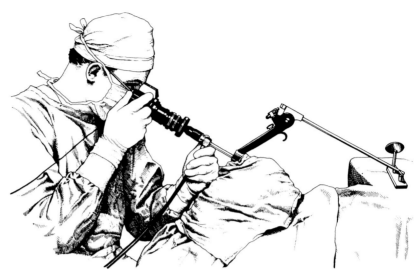

Figure 21. *Laryngeal photography using a rigid telescope.*

laryngoscope. The surgeon is now able to work with both hands (Figure 22). A beam splitter interposed in the microscope optics permits use of an observer tube (Figure 22) and documentation using still photography, cinephotography, or a video camera. Once positioned, the microlaryngoscope is supported by a self-retaining laryngoscope holder, the foot of which rests on a Mustard table (Figure 23).

Microlaryngoscopy and Laser Surgery. The carbon dioxide laser is a recent development for microsurgery in the larynx and upper airways. The microscope with the laser attached (Figure 24) is positioned so that there is absolutely clear access through the mouth of the laryngoscope. The laser beam allows precise destruction or excision of various lesions with minimal trauma to surrounding tissues.

The method is useful in the treatment of dysplasias, premalignant

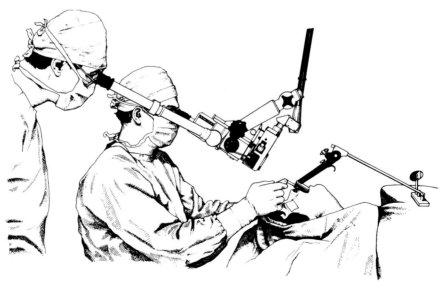

Figure 22. *Microlaryngeal surgery using a self-retaining laryngoscope holder. A beam splitter in the microscope allows use of an observer tube.*

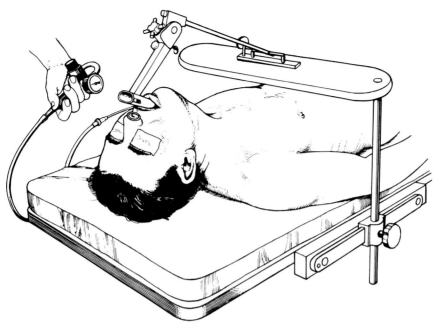

Figure 23. A Mustard table supports the laryngoscope and is firmly attached to the operating table.

conditions, and small invasive malignancies in the larynx. The laser can also be employed in the treatment of congenital and acquired webs or stenoses, and of some hemangiomas, lymphangiomas, and granulomas. Other endolaryngeal procedures, such as arytenoidectomy or removal of benign tumors and cysts, may also be performed with the laser. For a difficult anatomical site, such as the laryngeal ventricle or the subglottic

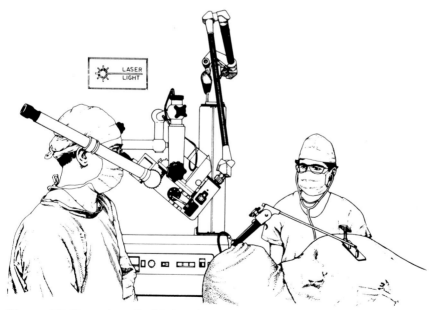

Figure 24. The carbon dioxide laser is attached to the microscope for use through the laryngoscope.

region, the laser beam can be reflected onto the lesion by small metal mirrors, and small metal "paddles" are used to protect the opposite vocal cord for work near the anterior commissure. It is particularly suitable for vaporization of laryngeal papillomas; multiple sites can be treated at one operation with due care to prevent scarring and web formation. Papillomas are vaporized precisely using the micromanipulator for constant visual control of the beam; there is virtual absence of bleeding, less reactive edema, and little postoperative pain. Cupped forceps, angled left, right, or upward, are sometimes required to remove residual papillomas from difficult areas after laser surgery and in conjunction with it. A laser beam with a small diameter provides an advantage in pediatric laryngology.

Precautions are required when laser energy is used. Combustible anesthetic gases are avoided if possible. With the inhalational technique of spontaneous respiration for infants and children, no anesthetic tube is necessary; but if a tube is used, great care must be taken not to ignite it. *The cuff of the tube should be filled with saline. If there is any possibility the tube has been burned or is about to ignite, all further laser treatment must be stopped and the tube removed immediately.* An attempt can be made to shield a tube with aluminum foil, and so-called "laser-shielded" tubes are available, but the protection is not always reliable. Metal endotracheal tubes cannot, of course, be ignited, but they are cumbersome. Laser energy is absorbed by moisture, and saline-soaked patties can be placed around the endotracheal tube to lessen the chance of inadvertent laser damage to the tube or the surrounding tissues. The surgeon should assume ultimate responsibility for safe use of laser energy.

The laser beam should not be allowed to reflect off shiny metal surfaces. A wet towel is used to protect the face and eyes of the patient. The eyes of all personnel in the operating room are safeguarded by having each person wear protective spectacles. The final switch of the laser is turned on only immediately before use and is turned off immediately when the laser is no longer required.

We prefer not to use the laser for vocal nodules, Reinke's edema, or small vocal cord polyps. These lesions can be grasped with a cupped forceps to exert traction on their base so that surgical removal can be achieved using curved or up-cutting scissors, leaving the nearby vocal cord mucosa intact. Cupped forceps and scissors give a more satisfactory and accurate removal down to the submucosal layer without injury to the basement membrane, vocalis muscle or the vocal ligament.

Technique in Infants and Children

Pediatricians, neonatologists, and pediatric surgeons are aware of the nature and incidence of upper respiratory tract airway problems in infants and children and the necessity for endoscopic investigation. In pediatric hospitals throughout the world the number of endoscopic examinations has increased, performed by the clinician best trained in monocular endoscopic examination and microlaryngeal techniques— the pediatric otolaryngologist.

In the investigation of congenital or acquired airway problems in infants, laryngeal examination alone is regarded as an incomplete assessment; diagnostic examination should include the tracheobronchial tree and in selected patients also the esophagus, nasal cavities, and nasopharynx.

The infant's larynx is higher, softer, more easily displaced, and more easily irritated and has a greater tendency to spasm than that of the adult. The smaller, more sensitive airways require instruments designed for pediatric use.

In the neonate, especially the sick premature infant, it is vital to conserve body heat and maintain hydration. Figure 25 shows diagnostic endoscopy in a newborn baby. Note the overhead heater, the insulation on the baby's head, the warm blanket, and the selection of different-sized instruments. Particular care of the delicate mucosa must be taken during endoscopy. There is no other time when teamwork among the nursing staff, the anesthesia team, and the endoscopist is so crucial to the patient's welfare. Improvements in equipment allow greater safety, but even so, the varying problems confronting the endoscopist demand that the operator be absolutely familiar with the complexity of the instruments and thus always be able to maintain complete control over their passage and manipulation.

DIRECT LARYNGOSCOPY

Direct laryngoscopy can be successfully and safely performed at any age, even in premature infants weighing less than 1,000 gm, but the delicate structures must be gently handled. The infant or child lies on his back on a regular operating table; there is no need for a head rest or for an assistant to hold the head.

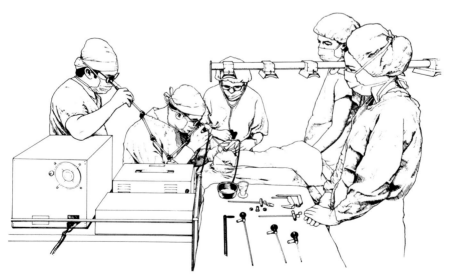

Figure 25. General view during endoscopy performed on a neonate. Note the careful monitoring by the anesthetist, the range of instruments available, and the overhead radiant heater.

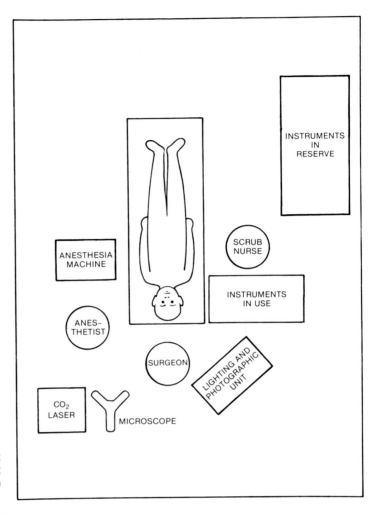

Figure 26. Suggested layout for personnel and equipment in the operating room for both adults and children.

Figure 26 shows a plan for the convenient layout of the instruments, lighting unit, microscope, laser, and anesthetic machine.

Direct laryngoscopy includes specific assessment of the oral cavity, base of tongue, pharynx, epiglottis, piriform fossae, larynx (including the appearance and movement of the vocal cords), subglottic region, and trachea. To provide for patients from premature babies to infants and older children, a range of endoscopes of different sizes and shapes are needed.

Anesthesia is induced with a face mask (Figure 27), which is removed as the administration of gases is temporarily suspended for application of the local anesthetic solution and, thereafter, during each phase of the endoscopic examination. A suitable-sized general-purpose laryngoscope (Figure 5) is chosen and the face mask and Guedel airway are temporarily removed (Figure 28). The laryngoscope is passed alongside the tongue in front of the epiglottis to view the valleculae and base of the tongue and then behind the epiglottis as the neck is extended to expose the larynx (Figure 29) by lifting the laryngoscope. A lever action is never used.

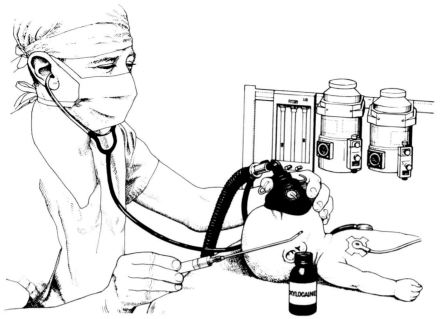

Figure 27. The anesthetist has induced anesthesia using a face mask and has prepared the local anesthetic solution to spray on the larynx.

With use of the finger or fingers on the anterior neck (Figure 30) for external manipulation of the larynx with gentle internal counterpressure from the distal beak of the laryngoscope, the structures can be rotated to better display the false cords, ventricles, and subglottic larynx.

In a patient whose larynx is difficult to expose and examine, a

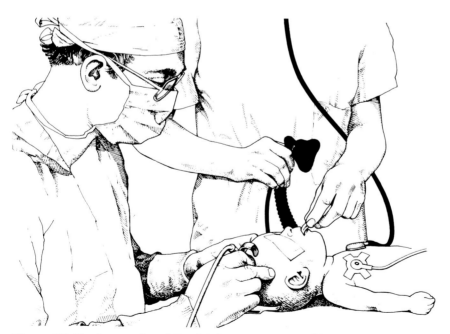

Figure 28. The face mask and Guedel airway are removed in preparation for direct laryngoscopy.

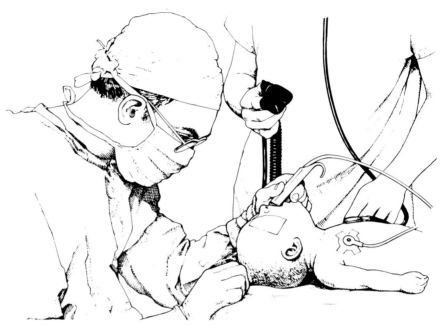

Figure 29. Direct laryngoscopy, during which the patient breathes room air.

special-purpose laryngoscope may be required. The *Holinger pediatric anterior commissure laryngoscope* and the smaller *Tucker-Benjamin slotted laryngoscope and subglottiscope* for infants are both slim laryngoscopes for use when it may be difficult to view the larynx. They are very helpful, for instance, in exposing the larynx for intubation or passage of a bronchoscope in patients with micrognathia or abnormalities of the middle third of the face. The anterior and posterior commissure and the interarytenoid region can be seen and displayed. Furthermore, by

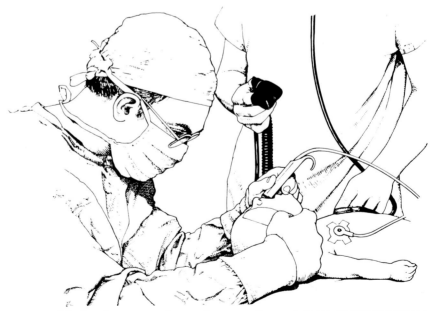

Figure 30. Gentle pressure from a finger on the neck helps display the larynx.

deliberately separating the vocal folds, the subglottic region is more satisfactorily exposed.

The face mask is replaced and anesthesia is deepened for the second part of the procedure, which entails a more detailed evaluation using rigid telescopes.

LARYNGOSCOPY WITH TELESCOPES

The face mask is removed and the general-purpose laryngoscope is again introduced. The 0° straight-ahead rigid Hopkins telescope (Figure 31) is used for a magnified image of the anatomical structures and the mucosa. With a 30° or 50° angled telescope the laryngeal ventricles, the anterior and posterior commissures, and the anterior subglottic region can be inspected in detail. An assistant can observe all phases of the endoscopy using the Wittmoser articulated optical arm (Figure 25). Photography can readily be undertaken through any of the telescopes.

As in adults, when used with either a hand-held laryngoscope or a laryngoscope placed in position and suspended, a telescope provides a more extensive and complete examination than is possible with an operating microscope. In fact, in many children the trachea, carina, and main bronchi can be clearly examined with a slim rigid telescope passed through the glottic opening and down into the tracheobronchial tree. In this way the laryngoscope is used to expose the larynx; to maintain the airway for anesthesia; and to allow tracheobronchoscopy to be performed, in some instances without the use of a bronchoscope. The alternative standard technique is to pass a bronchoscope for tracheobronchoscopy, first with the naked eye and then with a telescope in the bronchoscope.

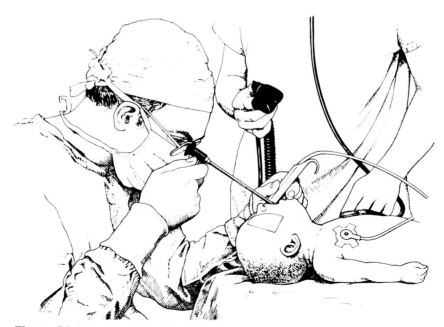

Figure 31. Laryngoscopy with rigid telescope.

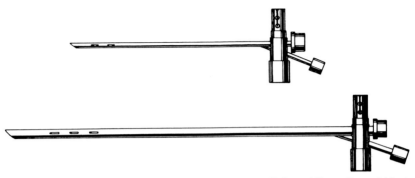

Figure 32. The smallest (2.5 mm) and the largest (6.0 mm) Storz Doesel-Huzly pediatric ventilating bronchoscopes.

TRACHEOBRONCHOSCOPY

The Storz Doesel-Huzly range of pediatric ventilating broncho-scopes (Figure 32) is satisfactory in design, function, and safety features. The complete range of rigid bronchoscopes includes instruments with internal diameters of 2.5, 3.0, 3.5, 4.0, 5.0, and 6.0 mm, available in different lengths and with adaptations to allow ventilation (Figure 33).

The size marked on the bronchoscope is misleading; it refers to the inside diameter of the lumen, not to the outside diameter (Table 1). It is crucial that a bronchoscope of suitable outside diameter be chosen so that there is no trauma as it passes the subglottic region. A bronchoscope of appropriate outside diameter and length is passed while the larynx is displayed using a laryngoscope (Figure 34), or alternatively the broncho-scope may be introduced directly without the use of a laryngoscope. The patient continues breathing spontaneously as anesthetic gases are administered through the ventilating bronchoscope (Figure 35). If the bronchoscope feels "tight," the next size smaller must be used to minimize subglottic trauma, which can create irritation and subglottic edema postoperatively.

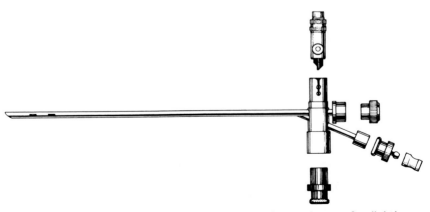

Figure 33. A "broken" view showing the various adapters for lighting and anesthesia.

Table 1. Sizes of Bronchoscopes

Size Marked on Bronchoscope (mm)	True External Diameter (mm)	Age Range
2.5	4.0	Premature to neonate
3.0	5.0	Neonate to 6 months
3.5	5.7	6 to 18 months
4.0	7.0	18 to 36 months
5.0	7.8	3 to 8 years
6.0	8.2	Over 8 years

If the bronchoscope is tight after it passes the glottic opening, the next smaller bronchoscope should be used to minimize subglottic trauma.

The tracheobronchial tree is examined, including the trachea, carina, main bronchi, and segmental and subsegmental openings, through 0°, 30°, and 70° telescopes (Figure 36). Abnormal secretions are aspirated into a trap bottle for examination and culture. The presence of any abnormal compression, collapse, stenosis, or other abnormality is noted. Biopsy of a mass is occasionally necessary.

ESOPHAGOSCOPY

Endotracheal intubation (Figure 37) is established to provide a secure airway for maintenance of anesthesia. An esophagoscope of suitable diameter and length is chosen from a range of pediatric instruments. The Negus pattern rigid instruments have a wide lumen, which is an advantage for open-tube manipulation, biopsy, removal of foreign bodies, and direct-vision antegrade esophageal dilatation.

The esophagoscope is passed through the right side of the mouth (Figure 38), advanced to the right piriform fossa, and moved to the midline, displacing and lifting the larynx forward to allow identification

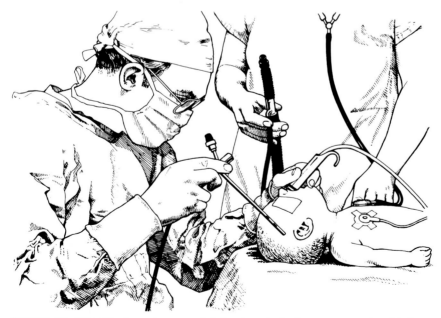

Figure 34. After the bronchoscope is introduced, the laryngoscope is withdrawn.

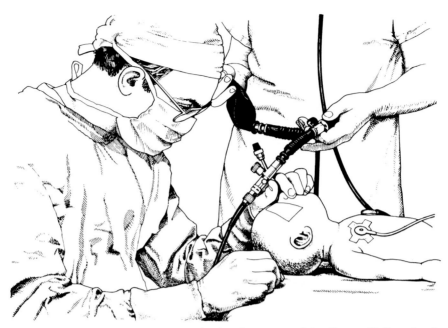

Figure 35. Attachment of the anesthetic adapter completes the ventilating circuit.

of the esophageal opening, which is guarded by the circular sphincter of the cricopharyngeus muscle. Relaxation of the sphincter allows the instrument to pass smoothly into the upper esophagus and down through the gastroesophageal junction into the stomach to reveal the gastric rugae. Elevation of the shoulders by an assistant's hand in the interscapular region assists passage of the esophagoscope to the lower end. In some patients, forward displacement of the membranous esophagotracheal wall may obstruct airflow in the trachea below the distal tip

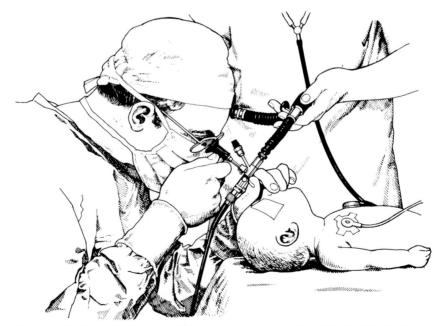

Figure 36. The tracheobronchial tree is examined with various telescopes.

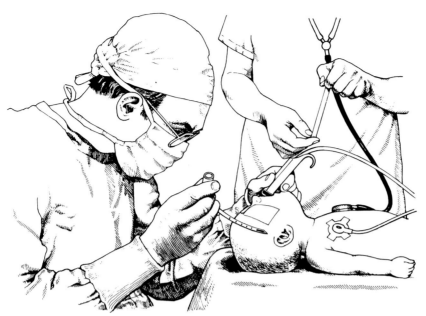

Figure 37. An endotracheal tube is introduced for esophagoscopy or examination of the nose and nasopharynx.

of the endotracheal anesthetic tube. Esophageal photography (Figure 39) is performed in a similar manner to photography of the larynx, but using a longer telescope.

Identification and withdrawal of an impacted esophageal foreign body is facilitated using appropriate grasping forceps and a rigid, open-tube esophagoscope with a larger-diameter, round lumen. Esophageal examination in gastroesophageal reflux allows biopsy or biopsies;

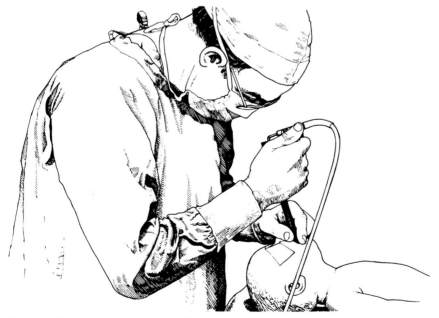

Figure 38. The esophagoscope is passed through the right side of the mouth before it is introduced into the upper esophagus.

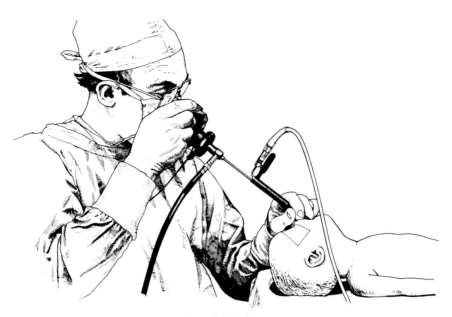

Figure 39. Photography through a rigid telescope.

histological examination may confirm a diagnosis of esophagitis or assist in the diagnosis of reflux changes in the mucosa of the lower esophagus. Antegrade dilatation of a stenosed area is best performed under direct vision through an esophagoscope with a wide-diameter, round lumen (Figure 40). Esophagoscopy may also be useful in identification of a congenital web or stenosis, compression by a pulsatile vascular ring, or indentation from an extrinsic cyst or tumor. The esophageal orifice of an H-type (more accurately called an N-type) tracheoesophageal fistula can be identified on the anterior wall by direct viewing or with a telescope.

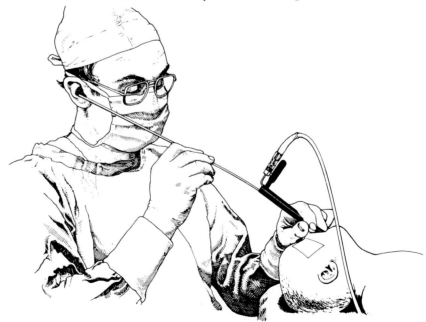

Figure 40. Esophageal dilatation with graduated bougies is performed under direct vision.

The tract runs obliquely downward and backward from the upper part of the posterior tracheal wall, and the esophageal orifice is seen, often with an inverted V appearance on the anterior wall of the upper third of the esophagus.

EXAMINATION OF THE NASAL CAVITIES AND NASOPHARYNX

Anesthesia is maintained via an endotracheal tube. The nasal cavities are examined using straight-ahead and 30° angled slim telescopes. It is important to decongest the nasal mucosa with a suitable agent in a measured dose to improve access and to minimize bleeding that might obscure the field. Neonatal nasal obstruction can be due to severe dislocation and deviation of the nasal septum, turbinate hypertrophy, encephalocele, cyst, or tumor or to congenital posterior choanal atresia. The latter is better seen from the nasopharyngeal aspect.

The self-retaining Dott-Dingman cleft palate gag (Figure 41) gives excellent access to the pharynx and indirectly to the nasopharynx and allows the use of both hands for inspection of the nasopharynx. A mirror or a 120° retrograde telescope can be placed behind the posterior edge of the soft palate with one hand, leaving the other hand available for aspiration of secretions, for biopsy, or any other surgical maneuver, for instance in the evaluation and surgical treatment of congenital posterior choanal atresia.

MICROLARYNGOSCOPY IN INFANTS AND CHILDREN

Microlaryngoscopy is often required in infants and children for surgical or laser treatment of papilloma, cysts, webs, stenoses, hemangioma, lymphangioma, or other conditions.

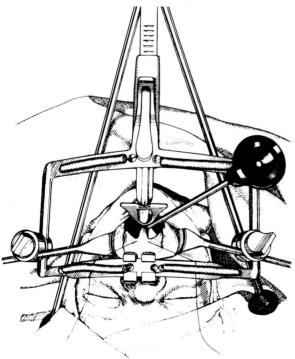

Figure 41. The soft palate is retracted by a single suture passed through the base of the uvula. The nasopharynx is inspected with a 120° telescope.

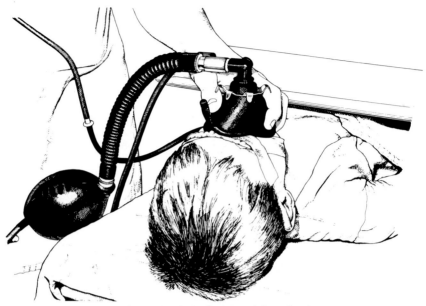

Figure 42. The level of anesthesia is deepened for microlaryngoscopy.

Anesthesia is deepened (Figure 42) to the required level. The face mask and Guedel airway are removed (Figure 43) to allow introduction of the *Benjamin pediatric operating microlaryngoscope,* which provides clear binocular vision for microlaryngeal surgery in children over 12 to 18 months of age. A smaller version has recently become available for use in treating infants and neonates.

The *Lindholm operating laryngoscope,* although designed for use in adults, can be used satisfactorily, without trauma, in most infants over 6 to 9 months of age.

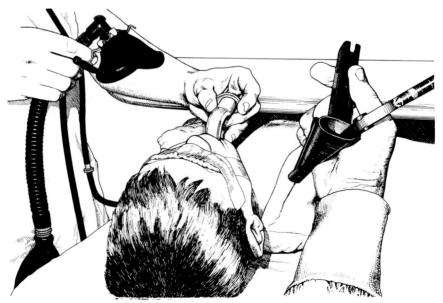

Figure 43. The face mask and Guedel airway are removed to allow the laryngoscope to be introduced.

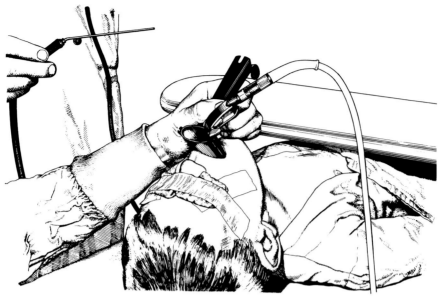

Figure 44. The laryngoscope is positioned and the metal cannula for anesthetic gases is ready to be placed in the wall of the laryngoscope.

The *Healy subglottiscope* has a limited application but is useful for microsurgery or laser surgery in the subglottic region in infants. Its narrow distal barrel separates and protects the vocal cords for treatment of subglottic or even upper tracheal pathology such as papilloma or hemangioma.

Anesthesia is maintained by insufflation of gases (Figure 44) through a metal cannula, in the wall of the laryngoscope. The position of the microlaryngoscope is adjusted, and a self-retaining laryngoscope holder

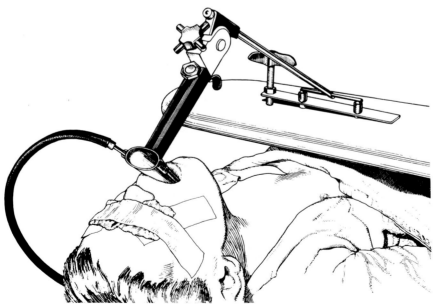

Figure 45. The self-retaining laryngoscope holder is positioned on the Mustard table.

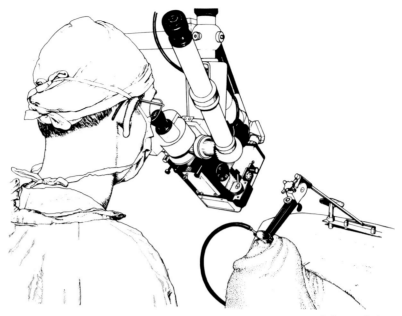

Figure 46. For endolaryngeal laser surgery the eyes and face of the patient are protected by a moist towel.

is positioned (Figure 45) for suspension laryngoscopy. The foot of the holder rests on the Mustard table over the chest of the patient. The same technique is employed for carbon dioxide laser surgery, with the precaution that the eyes and face of the patient are protected by a wet towel (Figure 46).

The same technique of photography as described previously can be used. The widest and best field is obtained using a Lindholm laryngoscope (Figure 47).

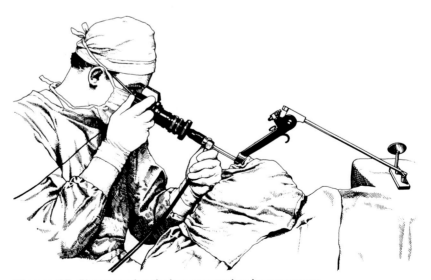

Figure 47. Photography during suspension laryngoscopy.

SPECIAL LARYNGOSCOPY TECHNIQUES

Difficult Laryngoscopy in Adults

A satisfactory view of the pharynx and larynx at direct laryngoscopy depends upon good general anesthesia, the choice of the correct laryngoscope, the skill and experience of the laryngologist, and a number of variable anatomical differences seen in individual patients.

It is not uncommon to have difficulty visualizing the anterior commissure in adults. A slim instrument such as the Holinger anterior commissure laryngoscope, the Benjamin slimline microlaryngoscope, or the Kleinsasser D laryngoscope is advantageous for direct vision and instrumentation. Alternatively, a 30° telescope will allow a precise but indirect view. Occasionally in thickset, muscular males with a broad neck, prominent incisor teeth, and a large epiglottis it is difficult to see any part of the larynx except the arytenoids or the posterior commissure. The slimmest laryngoscope should be passed at an angle through the side of the mouth, the suspension arm slowly opened, and observation made through an angled telescope to permit a more adequate examination. Very rarely the anatomical difficulties are so great that a view of the larynx can be obtained only by using a short open-tube bronchoscope or a child's short esophagoscope.

The difficulties with direct laryngoscopy apply equally to exposure of the glottic opening for passage of an endotracheal anesthetic tube. Many techniques have been described, including "blind" pernasal intubation, sliding an endotracheal tube placed over an "introducer" or a long rigid telescope, or alternatively using a flexible fiberscope that has already been passed into the trachea. A number of other ingenious techniques have been described.

Complete preoxygenation for at least 5 minutes before anesthesia is commenced is a valuable technique to safely extend the time available for instrumentation and intubation.

There will be difficulties with intubation and laryngoscopy in patients who have burn contractures of the neck; swelling of the floor of the mouth; micrognathia; macroglossia; prominent, unstable, or reconstructed teeth; restricted opening of the mouth; temporomandibular joint fixation; limitation of cervical spine extension; or a large mass such as a cyst, abscess, or tumor already compromising the airway and making instrumentation with a laryngoscope hazardous. In some cases of laryngeal or supralaryngeal obstruction it is safest to establish a tracheotomy using local anesthesia before dealing with the primary pathology.

Difficult Laryngoscopy in Infants

The Pierre Robin syndrome or midfacial skeletal abnormalities such as Treacher Collins syndrome, Apert's syndrome, or Crouzon's syndrome are often the cause of oropharyngeal airway obstruction in infants. Laryngoscopy is necessary only when the possibility of other congenital airway anomalies needs to be excluded or when endotracheal intubation is undertaken to provide a temporary artificial airway.

Laryngoscopy can be an extremely difficult technical procedure and in newborns is usually best done without general anesthesia but with cooperation between the anesthesiologist and the endoscopist. The anesthesiologist monitors the pulse rate, electrocardiogram, and arterial oxygen saturation and is prepared to administer anesthesia once an endotracheal tube or a bronchoscope has been successfully passed into the trachea. Laryngoscopy is less difficult using the Holinger pediatric slotted anterior commissure laryngoscope or the smaller Tucker-Benjamin slotted laryngoscope for premature or small babies. These special-purpose slim laryngoscopes give a view of the larynx in infants when others do not.

Laryngoscopy can be difficult also in infants with micrognathia; macroglossia; lymphangioma or hemangioma of the oropharynx; or aberrant thyroid tissue, which is most often seen as lingual thyroid but sometimes is found elsewhere in the pharynx. Mucous retention or ductal cysts, dermoid cysts, saccular cysts, thyroglossal duct cysts, peritonsillar and other pharyngeal abscesses, teratomas, chordomas, and other tumors each present particular problems.

Biopsy

Biopsy of a laryngeal lesion is necessary for histopathological confirmation of a diagnosis.

When the lesion is uniform and clearly delineated, a single representative biopsy may be taken, preferably from the edge so that it straddles the margin of the tumor and the apparently normal nearby tissue; a biopsy from this site may assist the pathologist to determine the presence of invasive cancer. All biopsy samples should be generous, taken with forceps with jaws 2 to 4 mm in diameter. At the same time prudence is required to avoid unnecessary violation of, or injury to, important anatomical structures such as the anterior commissure, vocalis muscle, vocal ligament, or the vocal process of the arytenoid cartilage. In cases of suspected malignancy adequate, representative, and multiple biopsies are important and sometimes take precedence over conservation of normal laryngeal structures. With some lesions, for example a small vocal cord polyp, the procedure is an excisional biopsy, whereas with others, for example a large malignant tumor, multiple biopsies carefully mapped and labeled according to anatomical site are required for evaluation of the site and extent of the tumor. Use of the laser for a small lesion may totally destroy it or distort the remaining tissue and so preclude a microscopic diagnosis. Therefore a small tumor, for example a suspected malignancy in the central part of a vocal fold, is better removed by excisional biopsy using cupped forceps and scissors than by using the laser.

Occasionally a diffuse submucosal swelling with intact mucosa requires a surface incision using a cutting instrument or a laser beam to provide access so that a deep biopsy specimen can be taken from the tumor itself.

Study of a frozen section of biopsy material is helpful when the necessity for further endoscopic or major extirpative surgery at the time of the biopsy depends upon the result. Making a frozen section is advisable in cases in which there is some doubt about adequacy of the biopsy; it makes certain that representative tissue has been taken to permit diagnosis. Where margins of resection need to be checked after endolaryngeal removal of a tumor, biopsy specimens for frozen section are indispensable to ensure that removal has been achieved.

Repeat biopsies at short or long intervals may be required in patients who have had radiation therapy or in those whose laryngeal mucosa shows premalignant epithelial dysplasia and cellular atypia. The time for the biopsies is indicated by changes in the voice and the appearance at indirect laryngoscopy.

Malignant Cervical Nodes with "Occult" Primary Tumor

A small number of malignancies present only as solitary masses in the cervical lymph nodes with no other symptoms or signs and are considered to be metastases from so-called occult or hidden primary lesions. This diagnosis is made only after a thorough search for a distant or local primary tumor. Needle aspiration of the involved node usually indicates the need for a search for the primary lesion by peroral panendoscopic examination of the nasopharynx, oropharynx, larynx, tracheobronchial tree, postcricoid region, and esophagus. This examination involves careful finger palpation of the floor of the mouth, tonsils, valleculae, and base of the tongue. An inconspicuous primary lesion may thus be seen, felt, or suspected. Biopsy specimens must be taken from all doubtful areas, including the nasopharynx, where "blind" biopsy sampling from the fossa of Rosenmüller can sometimes lead to discovery of an otherwise undetectable tumour.

The search for the undetected primary site should continue even after treatment of the cervical nodes has been undertaken.

Cricoarytenoid Joint Mobility

The differentiation of a paralyzed vocal fold from a fixed arytenoid cartilage is fundamental; the management may be very different.

An immobile vocal cord is usually due to vocal cord paralysis but is occasionally due to fixation of the cricoarytenoid joint, and sometimes both paralysis and fixation may be present in the same larynx. Mobility of the arytenoid cartilage on the articular facet of the cricoid cartilage can be limited in patients with generalized arthropathy; this is most often related to rheumatoid arthritis, but it can also occur in some of the other generalized connective tissue disorders or can be associated with arthrogryposis multiplex congenita in children. Mobility may also be limited when the joint has been involved by prolonged intubation trauma with posterior glottic stenosis, external trauma, dislocation of the arytenoid, malignant infiltration, postradiation changes, or chronic perichondritis or after prolonged vocal cord paralysis.

Visualization of a nonmoving vocal cord at indirect examination may lead to an erroneous diagnosis of "vocal cord paralysis" when the problem is really a fixed cricoarytenoid joint. Passive mobility of the joint can be assessed only during direct laryngoscopy with the patient under general anesthesia, with care taken that the position of the laryngoscope blade does not restrict the movement of or displace the arytenoid cartilage. A blunt instrument or suction tip placed against the medial surface of the arytenoid just behind the vocal process is used to move the arytenoid and test lateral displacement. The posterior glottic opening should be widened when a normally mobile arytenoid is moved laterally.

Teflon or Gelfoam Injection

Unilateral vocal cord paralysis causes a breathy, weak, and husky voice, at first with aspiration and an ineffective cough. In cases of recent onset in which there is no hope of recovery, for example mediastinal metastases involving the recurrent laryngeal nerve, or in cases of unknown cause with continuing paralysis for 12 months or more, Teflon paste can be injected. It is used as a filler material in the paralyzed hemilarynx and is the simplest and probably the most effective procedure available. As an alternative, Gelfoam paste can be used before 12 months has elapsed when there is no certainty that the paralysis is permanent and when temporary rehabilitation of glottic competence is desired. Gelfoam causes minimal tissue reaction and is used in cases in which it is desirable for the patient or the surgeon to know the effect of vocal cord injection to justify proceeding later to Teflon injection. The beneficial effect of Gelfoam paste lasts 5 to 10 weeks while it is metabolized and gradually absorbed; as the hemilarynx returns to its preinjection state, the manifestations of the vocal cord paralysis return. When longer rehabilitation is desired, Gelfoam paste can be injected a second or even a third time to restore satisfactory function temporarily while the months pass and a decision can be made about using Teflon.

The injection technique is the same for Gelfoam and Teflon paste. The aim is to partly fill the hemilarynx and displace it to the midline so that the contralateral, functioning vocal fold can adduct to meet it and produce a satisfactory and effective voice.

Local anesthesia has usually been advocated for the injection procedure, because the effect on the voice can be judged during the procedure and used as a guide to the amount to be injected. However, for the last 5 years a relaxant general anesthetic technique has been employed using jet ventilation by means of a Benjet tube, which lies relatively unnoticed in the posterior commissure, causing no laryngeal displacement or distortion and therefore not interfering with accurate injection. This technique of general anesthesia is more comfortable for the patient, is less stressful for both the patient and the surgeon, and is recommended as an excellent alternative to local anesthesia.

There are some important points to be considered in the technique of injection. Cricoarytenoid joint movement *must* be normal to achieve an optimal result. A laryngoscope is used to separate the false cords and push the posterior part of the ipsilateral false cord laterally to expose the floor of the posterior part of the laryngeal ventricle. A high-pressure injection "gun" is used with a 19-FG, 20-cm needle, which is introduced as far laterally as possible just inside the lamina of the thyroid cartilage and lateral to the vocal process of the arytenoid and therefore between these two cartilagenous structures (see Figure 372). Sufficient paste is delivered, one click at a time, until the vocal fold reaches the midline. The first, most important, and often only site of injection is in the posterior lateral hemilarynx, but in selected cases a second, smaller injection in front of the first may be needed. If at any time a bulge appears in the subglottic region, further injection is stopped until the needle is withdrawn a little. After sufficient paste appears to have been injected, the succinycholine intravenous infusion is stopped and jetting ceases as spontaneous respiration begins. Brisk vocal cord movement soon returns (see Figure 373) and a judgment can be made about the adequacy of the filling and whether a further injection is necessary. It is often not possible to close the posterior "respiratory" part of the glottic opening. If the laryngologist errs at all, he or she should err by placing too little rather than too much paste. Each patient needs to be informed that a second injection might occasionally be found necessary some months later.

Errors of technique (see Figures 374 to 378) include using too much paste, misplacement anterior to the vocal process, and placement too close to the edge of the vocal fold or too deep in the subglottic region. Granuloma formation occurs when Teflon is too close to the mucosal surface.

Multiple Respiratory Papillomatosis

Repeated surgical removal with forceps or preferably with the carbon dioxide laser remains the best form of palliative management for papillomas in the upper respiratory tract. Many of the patients requiring repeated treatment are infants or children; overall two thirds are patients under 15 years of age and one third are older patients.

Particular care should be taken to maintain the airway during induction of anesthesia for the initial examination in patients who have suspected or known papillomas despite the fact that airway obstruction may not be apparent or may appear to be minimal at preoperative assessment. Progressive obstruction may occur as the depth of anesthesia is increased, and it is safest to commence anesthesia in the operating room with an endotracheal tube, a laryngoscope, and a bronchoscope readily available.

At the first examination precise and comprehensive panendoscopic assessment of the upper aerodigestive tract is necessary to ascertain the location and spread of the tumors. Laryngoscopy at the first examination should remove a large bulk of the growths on one side of the larynx to improve the airway and for histopathological confirmation of the diagnosis.

The aim of treatment in obstructive cases is to maintain a clear airway at least sufficient to avoid a tracheotomy. The aim of treatment in nonobstructive cases is to achieve "control" by the eradication of all papillomas; most patients require operation at intervals of 2 to 6 months, but the rate of growth and the frequency of operation vary from patient to patient.

The carbon dioxide laser with variable spot size is advantageous in papilloma removal and is used in almost every case. Often it is used in conjunction with angled cupped forceps to remove papillomas more satisfactorily from within the ventricle, where access and visualization are limited. Care must be taken to avoid injury to normal laryngeal structures, as the potential for adhesions and web formation at the anterior commissure is high, especially in inexperienced hands.

Techniques to minimize web formation are important, and include strict limitation of surgery to one side, especially at the anterior commissure; use of small cupped forceps, which allow a "feel" of the underlying tissues that is not obtained with laser surgery; use of a laryngoscope to separate the false cords and to some extent the true cords to allow more precise surgical removal; external finger pressure to manipulate the papilloma into a direct line for laser treatment; and sometimes use of a metal mirror to bounce the laser beam into otherwise inaccessible anatomical areas such as the ventricle, where access and visualization are limited. When the tumors cannot be completely removed at one operation the surgeon, patient, and parents should accept the need for repeated operations. It is difficult to define "too much" surgery at one operation, but discretion on the part of the surgeon will minimize overzealous treatment.

Subglottic or upper tracheal lesions are treated with a direct laser beam where possible, using the laser coupled to the operating microscope. In adults the "slimline" microlaryngoscope or in children the subglottiscope can be used to separate the vocal cords and expose the operative site. Where lesions are in the middle or lower trachea or the bronchi, the bronchoscopic coupler for microsurgical application of the carbon dioxide laser is used.

Trauma Due to Endotracheal Intubation

Endoscopic evaluation using an open-tubed laryngoscope and rigid telescopes, with the patient under general anesthesia, enables the laryngologist to identify the changes that occur in the larynx during prolonged endotracheal intubation whether in adults, children, or infants. Laryngeal damage is caused by pressure from the wall of the tube exceeding capillary perfusion pressure and producing a localised ischemic injury.

There are certain sites of predilection for damage, and attention must be directed to the medial surfaces and vocal process of the arytenoids, the cricoarytenoid joints, the posterior commissure, and the subglottic region including the anterior surface of the cricoid lamina. It is noteworthy that the supraglottic region and the anterior commissure seldom have significant involvement; edema of the vocal folds and edematous prolapse of the mucosa of the ventricles may be prominent, but these changes subside quickly and leave no permanent sequelae.

After even a few hours of intubation, laryngoscopy with image magnification reveals mucosal hyperemia and reactive edema. Thereafter ischemic pressure necrosis, typically recognized as epithelial erosion and ulceration, is the fundamental lesion from which further complications occur. If the endotracheal tube is removed at this stage of minor or moderate epithelial erosion, healing by primary re-epithelialization will usually occur.

After several days of intubation, granulation tissue will form at the vocal process of the arytenoids, where the mucoperichondrium is thin and tightly adherent. If the tube is removed at this stage, these more extensive lesions begin to heal by secondary intention with granulation tissue formation; when this is exuberant, a localized granuloma may proliferate. In a few cases granulomatous changes at the vocal process of the arytenoid persist weeks later, having formed mature intubation granulomas.

With continued presence of the endotracheal tube, confluent ulceration and deep stromal necrosis extend the degree of perichondrial and cartilage involvement. Ulceration to cartilage within the cricoid can stimulate an attempt at healing, with eventual maturation of fibrous tissue; this can progress to an acquired subglottic stenosis with or without chronic perichondritis, edema, and granulation tissue.

Posterior glottic stenosis is a serious complication and occurs when scarring, contracture, and fibrosis forms a band or web in the posterior commissure following pressure necrosis, ulceration, and erosion of perichondrium and cartilage. The vocal cords cannot be abducted where there is posterior glottic stenosis.

Specific lesions seen for assessment at endoscopy can be classified into two groups: first, changes seen in the intubated larynx, and, second, changes that occur following successful extubation but present weeks or months later.

CHANGES IN THE INTUBATED LARYNX

Early Nonspecific Changes. Irritative hyperemia and edema at the vocal process of the arytenoid (see Figure 213) are the earliest focal changes seen, and they are soon associated with surrounding surface mucosal ulceration.

Granulation Tissue. Tongues of granulation tissue (see Figures 215 and 223) form consistently on each side from the vocal process of the arytenoid and pass anteromedially, encircling the anterior surface of the endotracheal tube. There is almost always natural resolution if the irritation of the endotracheal tube is removed; no attempt to remove these tongues of granulation tissue surgically is necessary. Rarely, if they join together across the midline an interarytenoid adhesion forms. In other cases, unilateral or bilateral mature intubation granulomas form and persist.

Ulceration. Ulceration occurs in the posterior larynx, in the interarytenoid region and on the anterior surface of the cricoid lamina (see Figures 222 and 225). Superficial ulceration will heal when the tube is removed, but deep ulceration implies a risk of later fibrosis and posterior glottic stenosis. This area is an important site for endoscopic evaluation.

Ulcerated "Trough." On removal of the endotracheal tube a linear, shallow, rounded "trough" ulcerating the medial aspect of the arytenoid cartilage and the cartilage of the cricoid with exposure of the crico-arytenoid joint may be seen on one or both sides (see Figure 226). This acute change implies later chronic dysfunction of the joint, and the ulcerated trough can subsequently be recognized in the extubated larynx as a healed "furrow."

It is important to monitor the progression of changes in prolonged intubation by endoscopic assessment at regular intervals. Where there is deep ulceration over large areas in the posterior commissure with erosion of perichondrium and bare cartilage exposure, there is a significant chance of serious chronic laryngeal damage. Unless intubation is to be terminated in the near future, within 24 to 48 hours, tracheotomy should be considered as an alternative airway to avoid serious long-term changes due to intubation.

CHANGES IN THE EXTUBATED LARYNX

Granuloma. Granulation tissue may persist at the site of maximum reactivity as unilateral or bilateral intubation granulomas (see Figure 234) at the vocal process of the arytenoid, where the mucoperichondrium attaches directly to the cartilage with an absence of a submucosal layer. A granuloma may occasionally be found in an atypical site, such as the anterior commissure (see Figure 235) or the subglottis (see Figure 236).

Nodule of Scar Tissue. Nodule formation is a further consequence of intubation trauma seen on the medial aspect of the arytenoid and is a change that has not previously been clearly described. Granulation tissue at the vocal process usually resolves, but occasionally it forms a mature intubation granuloma, and in other cases a raised, more or less healed fibrous area covered by mucous membrane remains as a firm, smooth, rounded intubation nodule.

Healed "Furrow." In some patients a narrow linear "furrow" can be identified in the weeks, months, or years after intubation trauma when the larynx is assessed with care and precision (see Figure 241). This furrow can be seen running in a craniocaudal direction on the medial aspect of the arytenoid and the cricoarytenoid joint and represents incomplete healing of the ulcerated "trough," which is seen in the intubated larynx in the acute phase. The furrow causes persistent and troublesome dysphonia, which some individuals complain of after prolonged intubation. It is common to see other minor but definite changes, such as chronic edema in Reinke's space of the vocal folds in these same individuals.

Posterior Glottic Stenosis. The posterior glottic region suffers most from ischemic pressure necrosis and ulceration. In minor cases healing will be complete without functional deficit. In severe cases, after extubation, incomplete healing of the ulcerated area leaves granulation tissue (see Figure 237) that matures to scar tissue over the following months and causes chronic postintubation posterior glottic stenosis (see Figures 238 to 240) with partial or complete fixation of the cricoarytenoid joints and limitation of abduction. Posterior glottic stenosis is often poorly assessed or missed altogether, confused with bilateral abductor paralysis; or said to be nonspecific "laryngeal stenosis," an indefinite and imprecise term.

A conservative approach to this serious problem is to divide the transverse fibrotic scar, which appears as a firm, thick web with or without a diaphragmatic edge. It can be divided with the laser or, more commonly, with a curved No. 11 scalpel blade on a long handle. The web is boldly and deeply divided from the subglottic region to the interarytenoid region deep enough that the tip of the scalpel blade can be felt on the cricoid lamina. The tissues partly spring apart, leaving a deep V-shaped notch so that the posterior commissure stenosis is "released." The patient has immediate, dramatic relief of airway obstruction, but subsequently the incision heals and stenosis recurs. Therefore, most patients require repeated division of their posterior glottic stenosis, as often as every 6 months or as seldom as every 2 years. Other, more complicated surgical procedures require thyrotomy for posterior laryngoplasty with or without arytenoidectomy.

Interarytenoid Adhesion and Fibrous Band. A transverse interarytenoid adhesion (see Figure 229) occurs where granulation tissue from each side falls together and heals after the endotracheal tube is removed. Failure to divide the adhesion allows it to mature to an interarytenoid fibrous band (see Figures 230 and 231) that has a triangular "glottic opening" in front of it and a smaller rounded opening behind it, so that the vocal cords are tethered to one another and abduction is prevented. The adhesion or the fibrous band can be divided simply with the laser or with small microlaryngeal scissors; the results with either method are excellent.

Ductal Cysts. Submucosal ductal retention cysts develop in the subglottic region in infants who have been intubated previously (see Figures 353 and 354). The presentation is with stridor several months after extubation, and laser excision is the treatment of choice.

Vocal Cord Paralysis. Unilateral and even bilateral vocal cord paralysis is well recognized as a complication of short-term or long-term intubation. The nerve damage is thought to be compression injury of the anterior ramus of the recurrent laryngeal nerve as it passes between the arytenoid and the laryngeal cartilages. Recovery usually occurs within 6 months.

Dislocation of the Arytenoid. This is sometimes found after blind intubation or when an introducer has been used in the endotracheal tube (see Figures 251 and 252). It more commonly affects the left arytenoid, since intubation is done through the right side of the mouth with the tube tending to go toward the left in the larynx. The patient has pain on swallowing and persistent hoarseness, and laryngoscopy shows a displaced arytenoid with limitation of movement of the hemilarynx. In the acute stage an attempt can be made to manipulate the cartilage into a normal position, but most patients present later with limited movement in the cricoarytenoid joint. Endoscopic arytenoidectomy is a successful method of treatment.

Subglottic Stenosis. Acquired subglottic stenosis is a common complication of prolonged intubation, especially in premature babies treated by assisted positive pressure ventilation via an endotracheal tube indwelling for days or weeks. Soon after extubation a thin membranous web (see Figures 232 and 242) may be detected or there may be a "soft" subglottic narrowing due to edema. Later a firm fibrotic subglottic stenosis (see Figures 242 to 245) may be found. In advanced cases generalised laryngeal fibrosis with advanced scarring and stenosis is seen (see Figures 247 to 250).

DIAGNOSTIC FINDINGS IN INFANTS AND CHILDREN

Specific findings at laryngoscopy in some congenital and acquired conditions require brief description.

Laryngomalacia

A diagnosis of laryngomalacia can be made confidently only on the basis of direct examination. The anatomical features of laryngomalacia may sometimes be seen during the initial laryngoscopy, but usually are more apparent later as the administration of anesthetic gases is discontinued toward the end of the procedure (see Figures 90 to 95). During this latter, final stage of anesthesia, oxygen alone is administered via a small-diameter tube introduced into the oropharynx through one nasal cavity. There is ample time to assess the dynamics of the glottic and supraglottic structures as well as the return of vocal cord movement. The distal tip of the laryngoscope blade is placed above and in front of the epiglottis while the return of muscular tone and movement is awaited.

The epiglottis in laryngomalacia usually has an abnormal shape, being tall, narrow, and folded upon itself so that its lateral margins lie close together. This omega-shaped epiglottis, when seen from behind with a 30° telescope, has a tubular appearance (see Figure 94). The aryepiglottic folds and arytenoids are tall, thin, and flaccid and they are sucked into the larynx on inspiration, with accompanying inspiratory stridor. During expiration they are blown upward and outward so that outflow of air is totally unimpeded. When the laryngoscope blade is placed behind the epiglottis on its laryngeal surface and above the vocal cords the aryepiglottic folds and arytenoids are splinted outward, collapse of the airway is prevented, and the obstruction and stridor is immediately corrected.

The cause of laryngomalacia is not known with certainty. The abnormal flaccidity of the supraglottic laryngeal tissues is probably a temporary physiological dysfunction which resolves spontaneously, usually in 6 to 18 months, but longer in some patients.

Vocal Cord Paralysis

Vocal cord paralysis in adults and older children is best diagnosed at indirect laryngoscopy. In infants and younger children the diagnosis is made at direct laryngoscopy using a technique of general anesthesia that retains vocal cord movement (see Figure 367). Care must be taken with the assessment of vocal cord movement in unilateral or bilateral paralysis in infants and children. It is easy to misdiagnose apparent vocal cord "paralysis" caused in reality by pressure from the laryngoscope blade producing immobility of one side of the larynx. Abduction, adduction, and active movement of the arytenoids are patiently observed using a telescope during the final stage of laryngoscopy, when anesthesia has been discontinued and muscular tone returns.

In bilateral paralysis there is a narrow glottic chink and the vocal folds are slightly edematous with pink, irritated edges (see Figure 370). There is no effective abduction on inspiration but the cords "move" very slightly with the inspiratory and expiratory air flow. The larynx will close, with adduction of the false cords and supraglottic tissues during coughing and laryngeal spasm.

Subglottic Region

The internal diameter of the subglottic region within the cricoid cartilage should be recorded in cases of suspected congenital or acquired subglottic stenosis in infants and small children. A convenient method is measurement according to the outside diameter of the largest bronchoscope, telescope, or endotracheal tube that passes comfortably.

Congenital subglottic stenosis (see Figure 121) is the third most common congenital laryngeal anomaly after laryngomalacia and vocal cord paralysis. The most common presentation of this abnormality is generalized circumferential stenosis of the cricoid cartilage, but the lumen may be eccentric with a large anterior lamina, an oval or elliptical shape, a large posterior lamina, or generalized thickening. Soft subglottic stenosis may be caused by submucosal mucinous gland hyperplasia and must be distinguished from a congenital subglottic hemangioma, ductal cystic disease, or acquired narrowing from submucosal fibrosis and/or granulation tissue. The latter is more likely in a patient who has an underlying congenital subglottic stenosis.

Congenital Subglottic Hemangioma

Congenital infantile subglottic hemangioma is a mesodermal nest of vasoformative tissue that presents as a mass which usually occupies the lateral subglottis, seriously narrowing the airway. Patients present at 6 to 12 weeks of life with inspiratory stridor, at first variable but later severe, persistent, and life-threatening. The appearance at laryngoscopy (see Figures 96 to 99) is sufficiently characteristic for an experienced observer to make a diagnosis without the need for biopsy, especially if there are associated cutaneous hemangiomas. The laryngeal lesion is usually localized to the subglottic region on one side as a fairly firm, compressible, pink or bluish lesion. In some instances there are bilateral lesions (see Figure 100) or there is an extension below the posterior commissure (see Figure 101). Biopsy may be performed where the diagnosis is uncertain, taking due precautions to maintain the airway in the unlikely event that there is excessive bleeding.

Congenital Laryngeal Web

Laryngeal webs are not common. Most congenital laryngeal webs are anterior at the glottic level (see Figures 109 to 116) and affect the vocal cords, but some are posterior glottic or subglottic. The major feature is an abnormal cry, which is weak, husky, or even absent. With larger webs there is respiratory distress and stridor. It is important to assess not only the anteroposterior dimension but also the thickness. The latter is usually best seen and assessed on a preoperative xeroradiogram (see Figures 111 and 115), but further information is obtained during laryngoscopy by examination of the glottic and subglottic region with angled telescopes. With larger webs there is often a substantial congenital subglottic stenosis.

A congenital interarytenoid web in the posterior larynx is rare and produces interarytenoid fixation (see Figures 118 to 120). An erroneous diagnosis of bilateral vocal cord paralysis may be made because normal abduction is prevented by the band of tissue. During anesthesia and endoscopy the airway is difficult to maintain and exposure of the endolarynx is difficult.

Tracheoesophageal Fistula and Esophageal Atresia

Symptoms relating to the airway and to the esophagus after surgical repair of esophageal atresia and tracheoesophageal fistula are often present in the postoperative period and may be due to tracheomalacia, bronchomalacia, tracheal stenosis, esophageal anastomotic stricture, esophageal reflux with or without aspiration, and occasionally recurrent or residual fistula. The indications for endoscopy are both diagnostic and therapeutic. The diagnostic indications include evaluation in a neonate before operative repair of fistula and atresia, diagnosis of an H-type fistula, assessment of the degree and extent of tracheomalacia, identification of a recurrent, residual, or second fistula, detection of the presence of an associated anomaly (for example, subglottic stenosis or vocal cord paralysis), evaluation of esophageal stenosis, esophagitis, or gastroesophageal reflux. Therapeutic indications include dilation of an esophageal stricture and removal of an impacted esophageal foreign body.

In a neonate suspected clinically of having a tracheoesophageal fistula with esophageal atresia, the large opening of the fistula is seen on the posterior wall of the trachea, usually in the midline but sometimes to the left of the midline (see Figures 129 to 132). After removal of secretions, accurate judgments can be made about the site and size of the fistula, whether the mucosa is soiled by gastric juice, and whether there are infected secretions. A narrow catheter can be passed via the bronchoscope through the fistula into the lower esophagus and left in place to enable the surgeon to identify the fistula quickly at thoracotomy. This endoscopic examination is not necessary in all cases but may be reserved for the atypical or complicated case, for instance an upper pouch fistula, a double fistula, or a fistula in a patient with known or suspected associated anomalies of the respiratory tract.

Endoscopic identification of an elusive H-type fistula or a recurrent fistula requires meticulous examination of the posterior wall of the trachea and the anterior wall of the esophagus with angled telescopes looking for the openings of the fistulous tract (see Figure 141). The tracheal orifice is usually in the cervical region of the trachea and is best seen with an angled telescope. The esophageal aspect has a characteristic inverted V-shaped orifice (see Figure 142), which also may be difficult to identify. After a few milliliters of saline have been instilled into the upper esophagus, positive-pressure ventilation of the trachea through the endotracheal tube while an esophagoscope is in place blows bubbles of air from the fistula. Endoscopic catheterization of the fistula with a fine catheter facilitates surgical treatment. Associated anomalies of the trachea and/or the esophagus are common and include congenital tracheal stenosis, tracheomalacia, and esophageal stenosis.

Endoscopy has its most significant and well-established place following repair of atresia with fistula in the management of patients with "respiratory distress," infection, obstruction, stridor, retention of secretions, barking cough, aspiration, atelectasis, cyanotic attacks, or apnea. In the past these features were loosely considered as "postoperative pulmonary complications." Tracheomalacia is the major factor in producing these symptoms; the patients have a characteristic brassy, "barking" cough. In severe cases stridor develops during the first 2 months of life. They may also have sputum retention, cyanotic attacks, and severe apneic episodes. These attacks of "reflex apnea" are aptly called "dying spells."

In tracheomalacia there is collapse, weakness, and instability of the tracheal wall; the tracheal cartilages have an indented half-circle shape rather than a normal horseshoe shape; and the posterior membranous wall is markedly widened so that during expiration it bulges forward into the residual lumen of the trachea (see Figures 137, 139, 140, and 165). This typical triad affects several centimeters of the lower trachea, sometimes also involving one or other stem bronchus.

In cases of repaired fistula the residual pouch is invariably seen in the posterior tracheal wall (see Figures 137 and 138) as a diverticulum varying in length from a few millimeters to 15 mm. Occasionally a suture or granulation tissue may be seen within it. If the distal bevel of an endotracheal tube passes into this residual pouch, it may be impossible to ventilate the patient. The tube must be withdrawn 1 to 2 cm and repositioned with the bevel rotated so that normal ventilation can be achieved.

When a significant esophageal stricture begins to form after surgical anastomosis, early endoscopic inspection and dilation gives the best results. It is easier to treat a stricture in the early stages than when it is firm and fibrotic. Direct-vision bougienage is performed from above using graduated dilators. In difficult cases, retrograde dilation with Tucker's bougies is preferable and is the method of choice for dilation of a resistant stenosis.

As the primary results of surgery for esophageal atresia improve, long-term problems become increasingly important. The dramatic nature of some of these troubles, especially respiratory complications, and the overall generally good progress and prognosis using the latest techniques of corrective surgery mean that the endoscopist is now a vital member of the team in the care of these patients.

Tracheomalacia

In tracheomalacia there is an intrinsic weakness of the tracheal wall (Figure 48). Thus tracheomalacia is distinct not only anatomically but pathologically from laryngomalacia, in which no such structural abnormality has been demonstrated.

A classification based on the known histopathologic and endoscopic changes is:

Primary
    In premature infants
    In otherwise normal infants
    In the dyschondroplasias (all rare)

Secondary
    With tracheoesophageal fistula
    With innominate artery "compression"
    To external compression by blood vessels, vascular ring, tumor, or
    congenital cyst

The clinical features of tracheomalacia range from mild to severe, depending upon the location, length, and severity of the abnormal airway segment. They vary according to the causes included in the classification outlined above. Specific clinical features are associated with each condition. In general they include wheezing, cough (often a peculiar barking cough), inspiratory and/or expiratory stridor, recurrent respiratory infections, difficulty clearing endobronchial secretions, hyperextension of the neck, and dramatic episodes of respiratory arrest often referred to as "reflex apnea" or "dying spells."

Primary tracheomalacia sometimes occurs in premature or very premature infants treated for respiratory distress syndrome by prolonged endotracheal intubation with assisted positive-pressure ventilation. It is evidenced either by difficulty in placement of the endotracheal tube to

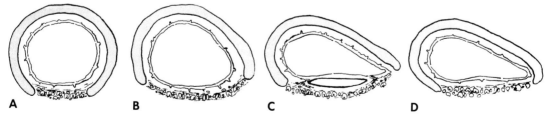

A   B   C   D

Figure 48. Basis for classification of tracheomalacia. Artist's reconstruction of transverse section of trachea based on known histologic and bronchoscopic changes. *A,* Normal trachea, with cartilage to muscle ratio of approximately 4.5 to 1. *B,* Trachea in primary tracheomalacia with cartilage to muscle ratio of approximately 2 to 1. *C,* Trachea in tracheoesophageal fistula showing residual pouch of fistula in posterior membranous wall. *D,* Deformed trachea in innominate artery compression with indented cartilage and wide posterior wall. (From Benjamin B: Tracheomalacia in infants and children. Ann Otol Rhinol Laryngol 93[5]:page 439, 1984.)

ensure reliable ventilation or in patients who, after extubation, have wheezing, stridor, and a barking cough and become prone to lower respiratory tract infection.

Primary tracheomalacia in mature infants who are otherwise normal presents in the first few weeks of life with unexplained respiratory distress, wheezing, cyanotic attacks, and inspiratory or expiratory stridor.

Bronchoscopy shows the typical lack of cartilagenous support, widened posterior membranous wall, and expiratory collapse and narrowing of the airway (see Figures 163 and 164). In severe cases prolonged intubation with positive-pressure assisted ventilation is necessary, sometimes for many weeks, but some patients ultimately perish.

Tracheomalacia associated with tracheoesophageal fistula has already been described (see Figure 165). At diagnostic endoscopy the typical triad is seen: indented semicircular tracheal cartilages, widened posterior membranous wall, and collapse and narrowing of the tracheal lumen in the anteroposterior plane.

Tracheomalacia can be seen associated with significant innominate artery compression (see Figures 145 to 148). The clinical features include inspiratory and sometimes also expiratory stridor, recurrent pneumonia or bronchitis, retained secretions, barking cough, attacks of atypical "croup," and attacks of reflex apnea and cyanosis.

The evidence of a structural abnormality of the trachea in innominate artery "compression" is inconclusive. At endoscopy it may be difficult to make the distinction between a normal "impression" and a pathological "compression" of the trachea where the innominate artery crosses. The endoscopic findings must correlate with the clinical features. The endoscopic observations in moderate or severe innominate artery compression are similar to those in tracheomalacia associated with esophageal fistula, with two notable exceptions. First, a shorter segment of the lower trachea is involved. Second, the associated findings of a wide posterior membranous wall with anterior bulging are not always present. It appears therefore that innominate artery compression causing significant clinical features can occur when the trachea is normal or when the trachea shows evidence of intrinsic tracheomalacia.

Tracheomalacia may be secondary to external compression by double aortic arch (see Figure 149) or one of its variants, bronchogenic cyst (see Figure 172) or other duplication cyst, teratoma, abscess, cystic hygroma, or hemangioma (see Figure 160). The clinical features will vary according to the causative pathology, and the secondary tracheomalacia presents as localized areas of soft, floppy tracheal cartilagenous wall that remain as areas of weakness after treatment of the primary pathology, for example after division of a vascular ring or removal of a bronchogenic cyst. It may be months or even years before this area of weakness becomes firm and the patient symptom-free.

Direct endoscopic examination with a rigid endoscope and telescopes, with the patient under general anesthesia, is the most reliable examination for a definitive diagnosis on which to base sound medical and surgical treatment of tracheomalacia. The diagnosis should not be made by exclusion; no amount of inferential supposition or "logical interpretation" of chest x-ray films thought to represent the inspiratory and expiratory caliber of the trachea can supply the information obtained at endoscopy.

Inhaled Foreign Bodies

Inhaled foreign bodies may lodge in the larynx or more often in the tracheobronchial tree. The highest incidence is in the second and third years of life. There is usually a history of a sudden coughing attack with choking, gagging, gasping, wheezing, cyanosis, or apnea lasting minutes or hours. With delayed presentation there is chronic cough, wheeze, a diagnosis of "unresolved pneumonia," or persistent changes in the chest x-ray with presentation days, weeks, or many months after the initial inhalation. Foreign body in the larynx is suspected when stridor, laryngospasm, husky voice, dyspnea, or inspiratory wheeze dominates the clinical picture.

With partial ball-valve obstruction of a main bronchus there is predominantly one-way inspiratory air flow with overdistention of the distal lung (Figure 49) and mediastinal shift. The x-ray changes vary according to the nature, size, site, and duration of impaction of the foreign body. A single negative chest x-ray is not sufficient to rule out the presence of a suspected inhaled foreign body. Fluoroscopic screening will reveal areas of overdistended lung, air trapping, and mediastinal shift.

A peanut is the most common foreign body (see Figures 193 and 194), and it is preferred that the fragment be removed in one piece. After it is located with a bronchoscope, secretions are cleared away and the fragment is gently grasped with peanut-grasping forceps to determine the degree of impaction and to obtain the "feel" of the peanut. The piece of nut can seldom be removed through the lumen of the broncho-

NORMAL AIR EXCHANGE   INHALED FOREIGN BODY IN RIGHT MAIN BRONCHUS

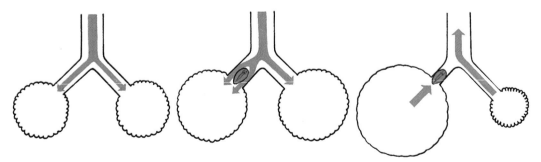

Inspiration and expiration have normal air flow each side.

During inspiration bronchial dilatation allows air flow past the foreign body and the lung fills.

During expiration bronchial constriction prevents air flow past the foreign body and the lung becomes overdistended.

Figure 49. The mechanism of ball-valve obstruction with an inhaled peanut. Where the presence of a suspected inhaled foreign body cannot be excluded, diagnostic endoscopy is indicated. Endoscopic procedures for removal of foreign bodies require a thorough knowledge by both surgeon and anesthetist of the techniques involved and of the potential hazards and complications. There must be a complete range of laryngoscopes, bronchoscopes, delicate grasping forceps, and ancillary equipment readily available.

scope; it must be grasped in the forceps and trailed after the broncho-scope as all three are removed together.

Removal of an inhaled foreign body in the tracheobronchial tree is a difficult procedure, but a foreign body in the larynx or subglottic area (see Figures 187 to 191) is often more difficult and the technique is critical. In some cases it may be safer to perform a tracheotomy to establish an airway below the site of impaction and airway obstruction before attempting to remove a difficult foreign body.

PRECAUTIONS, POSTOPERATIVE CARE, AND COMPLICATIONS

With reasonable care, experience, and attention to detail, anesthesia and endoscopy are associated with minimal morbidity.

Gentle technique, avoidance of endoscopic or laser trauma, and judicious use of a postoperative moist atmosphere for some pediatric patients are the principles followed to minimize postoperative edema, stridor, and respiratory distress.

In a neonate, especially a sick or premature one, meticulous care is required to avoid undue trauma during transport to the operating room and from excessive handling. It is vital to conserve body heat and maintain hydration. Particular care of the delicate mucosa must be taken during endoscopy. There is no other time when teamwork among the nursing staff, the anesthesia team, and the endoscopist is so crucial to patient welfare (Figure 25).

Complete preoperative assessment by the anesthetist and the surgeon should prepare them for any particular problem that might arise. The chest x-rays and the lateral airway x-ray or tomograms of the larynx should be readily available for reference. Review of any respiratory difficulty, anatomical features affecting airway maintenance or intubation, the effect of the patient's general health, and hydration is mandatory.

In those adults in whom there is pre-existent airway obstruction, anesthesia and endoscopic instrumentation may precipitate total obstruction and should therefore be attempted only if the diagnosis cannot be made in any other way or if endoscopic or surgical treatment of the obstruction is necessary. When such a problem is anticipated, anesthesia is started in the operating room with the endoscopic instruments functional and with instruments for a tracheotomy readily at hand.

Each piece of equipment must be in good order and checked before the procedure is started. Reliable suction must be available at all times.

Perhaps the most critical situation arises when partial airway obstruction suddenly becomes total. This may occur during induction of anesthesia or commencement of instrumentation in the presence of a large lesion in the larynx or pharynx. The x-ray should have revealed the presence of such a problem before it occurred, so that the surgeon should be fully prepared, for example, to decompress a cyst by sucking out its contents or by incising it or to pass an endotracheal tube or a bronchoscope around and past a supraglottic mass or tumor.

Irritation and edema due to inflammation or trauma from endoscopy or anesthesia can cause rapid swelling in the subglottic space in infants and children, especially if there is pre-existing airway obstruction. This problem requires gentle handling; excessive manipulation, passage of too large a bronchoscope, and prolonged and unnecessary manipulation must be avoided.

Other factors of importance include:

- Avoidance of unnecessary respiratory depression by injudicious administration of drugs, including premedication
- Vigilance in anticipating troublesome situations
- Prudent selection of instruments that will cause minimal trauma
- Careful handling of tissues already vulnerable to edema or bleeding
- Care in minimizing mucosal trauma with as little disruption as possible of the mucociliary mechanism of the respiratory tract
- Optimal humidification of the inspired air
- Adequate systemic hydration to maintain circulating blood volume where necessary by intravenous infusion of fluids
- Aspiration of secretions and blood during and at the completion of the examination
- Adequate facilities in a fully equipped recovery ward for recognition and treatment of potential complications
- Ready availability of expert medical resuscitation at all times

At the completion of the surgical procedure, care must be taken that the patient has recovered muscular tone and can support his or her own airway and that aspiration of secretions and blood is no longer required before the patient is returned to the recovery room.

Each and every endoscopic examination is necessarily traumatic in some degree because of the instruments passed, the trauma to the mucosa of the upper and lower respiratory tract, the drying effect of the anesthetic gases and atropine, and in small babies the loss of body heat and the actual handling of the child.

In infants and children the most common and most significant complication of diagnostic endoscopy is trauma in the subglottic region of the larynx caused by excessive manipulation, passage of too large a bronchoscope, or repeated manipulation. The result in the immediate postoperative period is subglottic edema, which manifests itself as croupy cough, stridor, and increasing airway obstruction. Should laryngeal edema occur or should it be a potential complication where the airway is already narrowed, adequate hydration of the patient, humidification of the inspired air, and if necessary administration of steroids in high doses are the methods of treatment. The efficacy of this use of steroids is unproven. The benefit of adequate humidification in helping to maintain a warm, moist respiratory mucosa should never be neglected. Drying of the mucosa of the upper respiratory tract and especially of the respiratory epithelium of the tracheobronchial tree has an adverse effect on the mucociliary mechanism and diminishes the efficiency of coughing. This may be compounded by trauma from instrumentation or by suction.

Other traumatic complications include loosening or dislodgment of teeth, laceration of the lips or gums, and bleeding from mucosal tears.

Positive-pressure ventilation, especially with the high-pressure jetting device, may produce pneumothorax or even laceration and disruption of the tracheobronchial tree. This is more likely to occur in the presence of diffuse pulmonary disease or even a minimal localized abnormality such as a small and otherwise inconsequential subpleural emphysematous bleb. The severity of the symptoms may be out of proportion to the radiological appearance of the pneumothorax. Prompt recognition of the cause of the respiratory difficulty and insertion of an intercostal catheter with underwater drainage is necessary.

It should be emphasized that adherence to careful technique reduces the incidence of complications to a minimum.

PART TWO

Atlas of
Clinical Illustrations

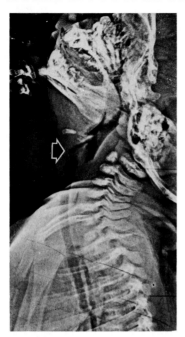

Figure 50. Lateral xerogram of the upper airways in a normal infant. The neck should always be in maximum extension. The nasopharynx, soft palate, oropharynx, epiglottis, arytenoids, and the extrathoracic and intrathoracic tracheal air column are seen. The laryngeal ventricle (*arrow*) is clearly seen with the false cords above and the true cords below.

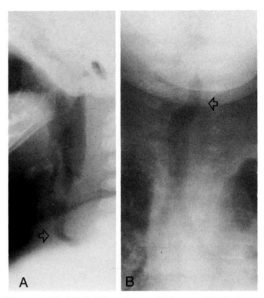

Figure 51. High kilovoltage (Kv) magnified views of the upper airways in an infant. *A*, The lateral view shows a kink in the upper trachea (*arrow*). *B*, The anteroposterior view also shows a kink in the upper trachea (*arrow*). Both appearances are normal variations often seen when the neck is not in extension.

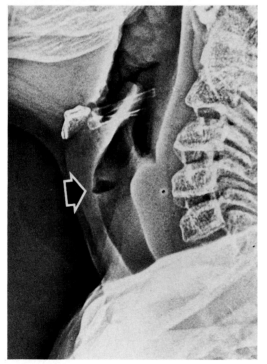

Figure 52. Lateral xerogram showing the laryngeal structures in detail. The valleculae, epiglottis, aryepiglottic folds, arytenoids, false cords, true cords, and subglottic region are seen. The ventricle (*arrow*) is distinctive.

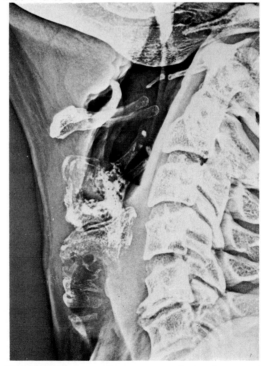

Figure 53. Lateral xerogram of the laryngeal region in an adult. Dystrophic calcification in the laryngeal cartilages prevents detailed evaluation. Lateral x-rays of the larynx are less useful in adults than in infants and children.

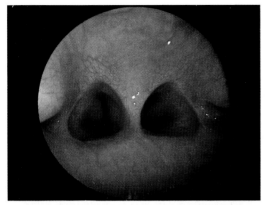

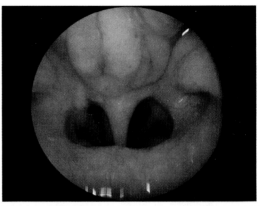

Figure 54. Normal nasopharynx of a newborn baby photographed with a 120° retrograde telescope. There is no adenoid tissue. The posterior end of the nasal septum, the posterior ends of the middle and inferior turbinates, and the eustachian tube openings are seen.

Figure 55. The nasopharynx of a 2-year-old child. The adenoid tissue is normal and the eustachian tube openings are seen.

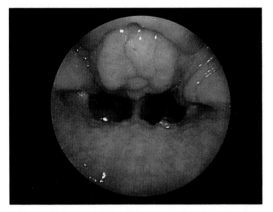

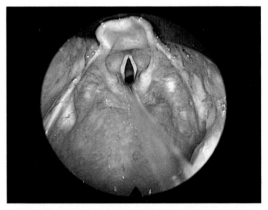

Figure 56. Large, healthy adenoids in a 4-year-old.

Figure 57. Adult larynx and laryngopharynx seen using the Lindholm laryngoscope. A jet anesthetic tube is in place.

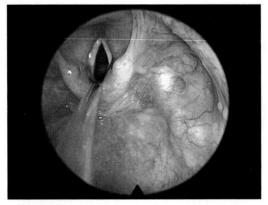

Figure 58. The right piriform fossa in the same patient.

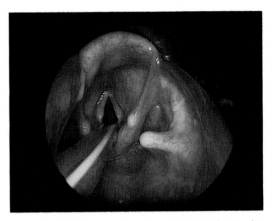

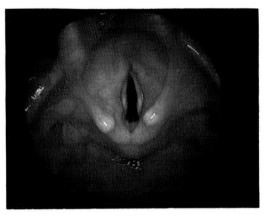

Figure 59. A prominent projection from the hyoid bone on the right lateral pharyngeal wall is not a sign of disease.

Figure 60. The normal adult supraglottic larynx and hypopharynx.

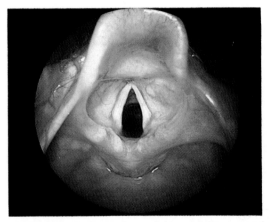

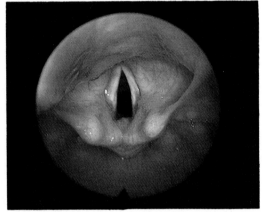

Figure 61. A closer view of the endolarynx and vocal cords.

Figure 62. The true cords, false cords, arytenoids, and aryepiglottic folds are normal.

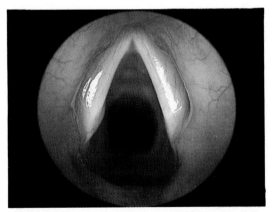

Figure 63. A close-up view of the vocal cords in abduction. The subglottic region can be seen.

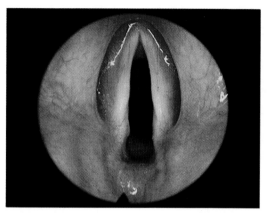

Figure 64. The upper surface of the true vocal cords, the posterior commissure, and part of the laryngeal ventricles.

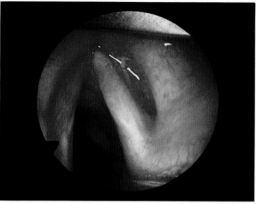

Figure 65. The right ventricle viewed with a 30° angled telescope.

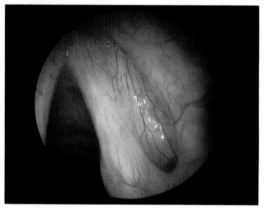

Figure 66. Close-up view into the right ventricle with an angled telescope.

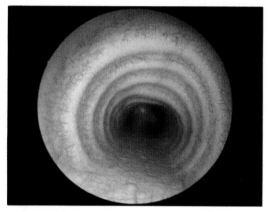

Figure 67. The upper trachea.

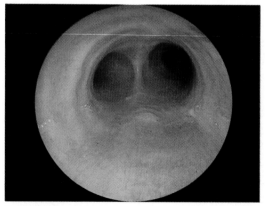

Figure 68. The carina, right main bronchus, and left main bronchus.

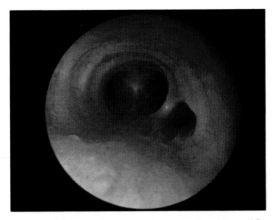

Figure 69. A right tracheal bronchus in a 10-month-old child. This is not an uncommon variation.

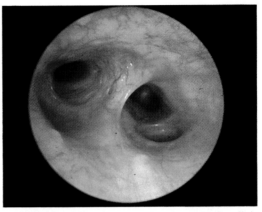

Figure 70. The upper division and lingular division of the left upper lobe and the openings of the left lower lobe bronchus.

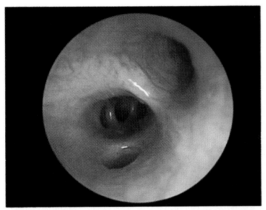

Figure 71. The opening of the right middle lobe bronchus and the segmental openings of the right lower lobe bronchus.

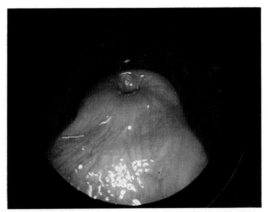

Figure 72. The circular cricopharyngeus muscle before passage of an esophagoscope.

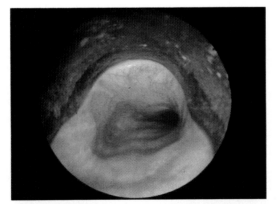

Figure 73. The normal esophagus showing the indentations of the vertebral bodies on the posterior wall.

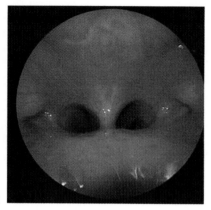

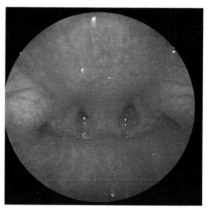

Figure 74. The normal neonatal nasopharynx (*A*) and bilateral congenital posterior choanal atresia in a newborn baby (*B*).

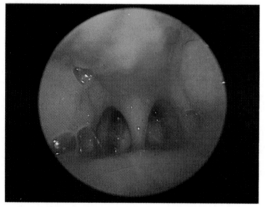

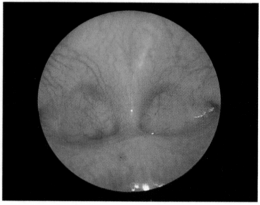

Figure 75. Bilateral choanal atresia. The site of bony atresia in this case is some millimeters anterior to the posterior end of the nasal septum.

Figure 76. Bilateral choanal atresia in another newborn baby. The plates of bone are near the plane of the posterior end of the nasal septum.

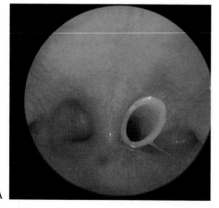

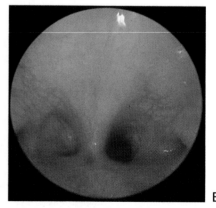

Figure 77. *A*, After removal of the abnormal atresia tissue, an endotracheal tube is left in situ. *B*, The appearance 2 weeks later. The atresia on the second side has been left for a second-stage operation.

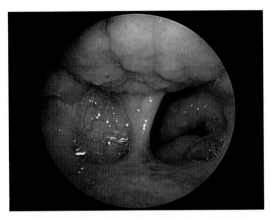

Figure 78. Unilateral posterior congenital choanal atresia.

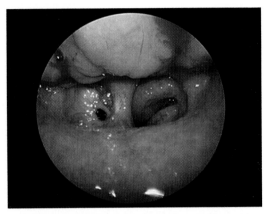

Figure 79. Partial stenosis due to reformation of some bone and fibrous tissue 12 months after transnasal surgical correction of congenital choanal atresia.

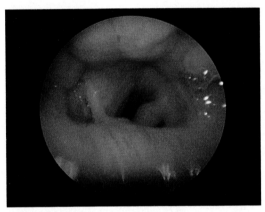

Figure 80. Unilateral choanal atresia with congenital stenosis of the posterior end of the nasal cavity. The CT scan will show this combined abnormality.

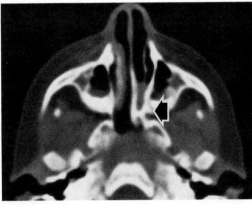

Figure 81. CT scan in unilateral choanal atresia, showing narrowing and stenosis of the posterior part of the nasal cavity and posterior bony atresia (*arrow*).

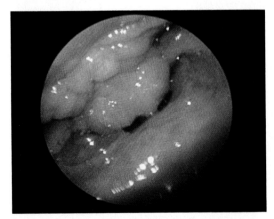

Figure 82. Enlargement of the adenoids causing severe obstruction of the nasopharyngeal airway.

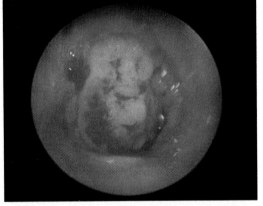

Figure 83. The anterior, hemorrhagic surface of the adenoids photographed with a telescope in one nasal cavity. There is complete obstruction.

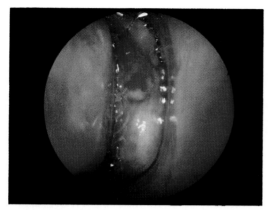

Figure 84. The anterior surface of a nasopharyngeal fibroma filling the posterior nasal cavity between the inferior turbinate and the septum.

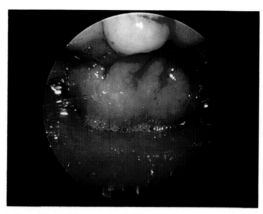

Figure 85. The nasopharyngeal view of a nasopharyngeal fibroma.

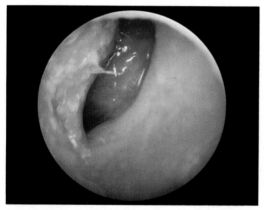

Figure 86. The smooth surface of a nasal encephalocele in the anterosuperior part of the nasal cavity in an infant.

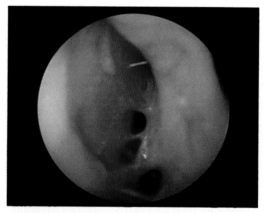

Figure 87. Prolonged use of indwelling tubes that were too large caused pressure necrosis and subsequent multiple bilateral nasal adhesions.

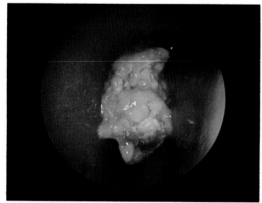

Figure 88. A rhinolith in the nasal cavity of a 10-year-old who had suffered from unilateral purulent nasal discharge for 2 years.

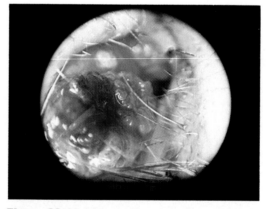

Figure 89. Multiple papillomas in the nasal cavity of a 16-year-old. There were no other papillomas in the upper aerodigestive tract.

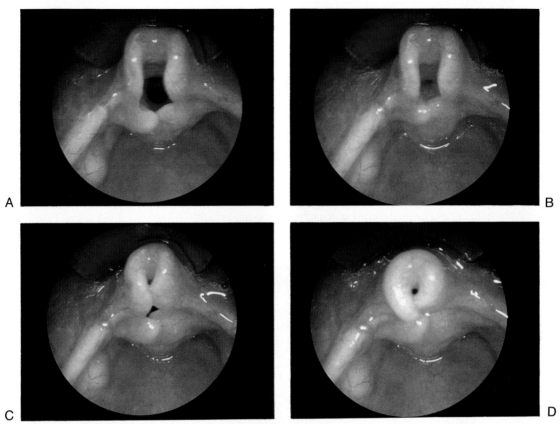

Figure 90. Laryngomalacia. *A*, Unimpeded expiration. *B*, Partial indrawing of the supraglottic structures producing stridor. *C*, Forward movement of the arytenoid cartilages, which further narrows the airway. *D*, There is only a tiny supraglottic laryngeal opening at maximum inspiration.

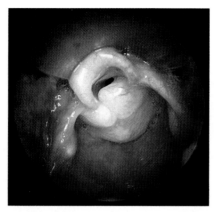

Figure 91. Forward movement of the arytenoids, especially on the right side, which occurs during inspiration in some forms of laryngomalacia. The blade of the laryngoscope has fixed the base of the epiglottis.

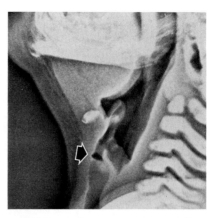

Figure 92. Lateral xerogram in an infant with laryngomalacia. The laryngeal ventricle (*arrow*) is foreshortened because of forward movement of the arytenoids.

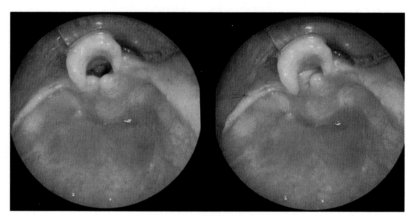

Figure 93. Tall, thin aryepiglottic folds and arytenoids that are sucked into the laryngeal introitus during inspiration.

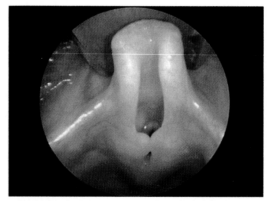

Figure 94. Through a 30° telescope the epiglottis is seen to be curled, tubular, and partly folded upon itself, so that its posterior margins lie close together.

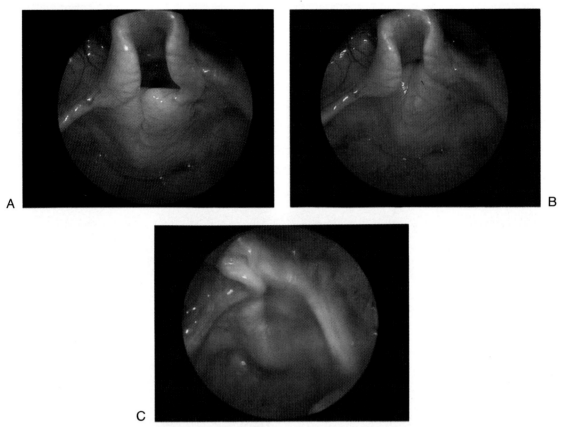

Figure 95. Changes during an inspiratory cycle. *A*, Expiration is unimpeded. *B*, During inspiration, the tall, "floppy," hypermobile arytenoids are sucked into the supraglottic opening. *C*, There is complete laryngeal obstruction with collapse and distortion of the supraglottic structures.

CONGENITAL LARYNGEAL HEMANGIOMA AND LYMPHANGIOMA

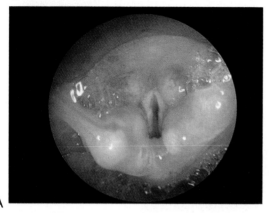

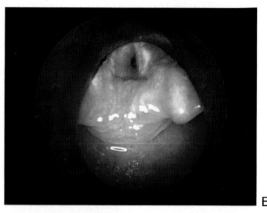

A

B

Figure 96. *A*, Diffuse submucosal hemangioma in the supraglottic tissues. *B*, When the laryngoscope pushes the vocal cords apart, a congenital subglottic hemangioma on the left side is revealed.

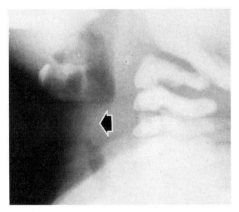

Figure 97. A circumscribed radiopacity in the subglottic region (*arrow*) on the lateral x-ray represents a subglottic hemangioma.

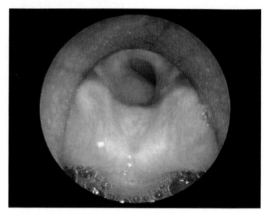

Figure 98. Congenital subglottic hemangioma under the posterior end of the left vocal cord and extending into the posterior commissure.

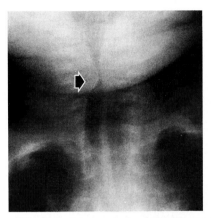

Figure 99. An anteroposterior high-Kv magnified image also shows a unilateral congenital subglottic hemangioma (*arrow*).

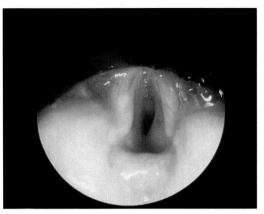

Figure 100. Bilateral congenital subglottic hemangiomas.

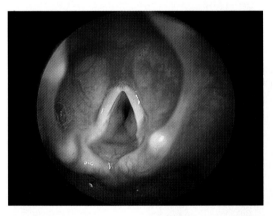

Figure 101. Congenital subglottic hemangioma presenting as three masses with severe obstruction.

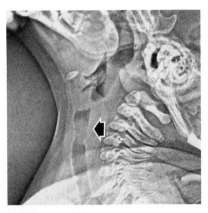

Figure 102. An oval, well-defined radiopaque mass (*arrow*) in the upper trachea of the 3-month-old child shown in the next endoscopic photograph.

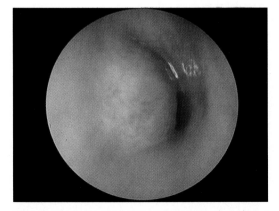

Figure 103. Endoscopic appearance showing a large hemangioma of the lateral wall of the upper trachea below the subglottic region, with almost total airway obstruction. It was removed surgically.

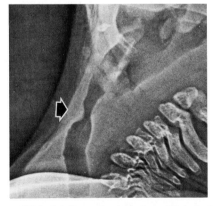

Figure 104. An 8-week-old baby with subglottic narrowing due to a hemangioma arising partly from the anterior wall of the upper trachea and partly from the posterior wall (*arrow*). See Figure 105.

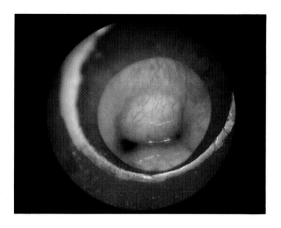

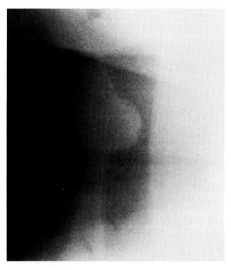

Figure 105. Large anterior and small posterior components in the subglottic and upper tracheal region.

Figure 106. Large, rounded mass on the anterior wall of the upper trachea. See Figure 107.

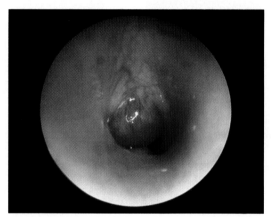

Figure 107. Endoscopy shows a large congenital hemangioma. The trachea was opened surgically, the mass was removed, and the trachea was closed. After 3 days of intubation, an uneventful recovery followed.

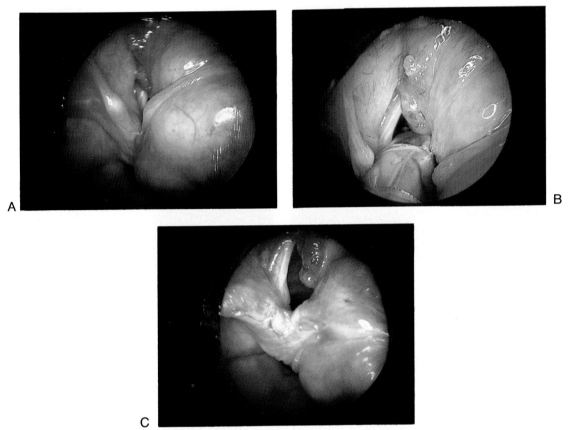

Figure 108. Three views of a cystic hygroma on the right side of the supraglottic larynx. *A*, Part of the left vocal cord, left arytenoid, and aryepiglottic fold can be seen. *B*, The airway obstruction has been overcome by passing an endotracheal tube wound with aluminum foil, preparatory to laser surgery. *C*, The tube has been removed, the airway is maintained by the laryngoscope, and further laser removal of the mass is about to begin.

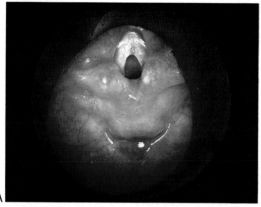
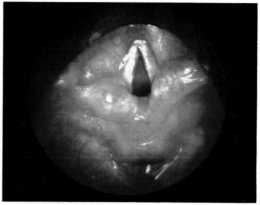

Figure 109. *A,* Small, thin congenital anterior glottic web in a baby who had no cry. *B,* Immediately after simple division of the web with microlaryngoscopy scissors. After recovery from anesthesia the baby had a normal cry.

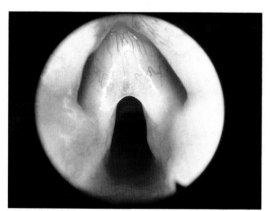

Figure 110. Medium-sized, thin congenital anterior glottic web in an infant with a weak cry.

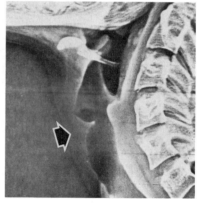

Figure 111. Lateral xerogram of a congenital anterior glottic web, clearly shows the thin posterior edge and the thick wedge of tissue anteriorly *(arrow),* which makes it difficult to obtain a satisfactory result from surgical treatment.

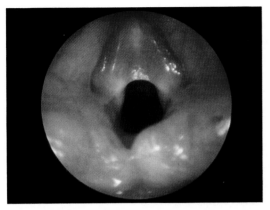

Figure 112. Endoscopic photograph of the web shown in Figure 111.

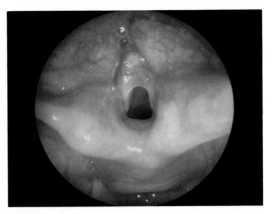

Figure 113. Medium-sized congenital anterior glottic web in a newborn baby with a weak cry but no airway obstruction.

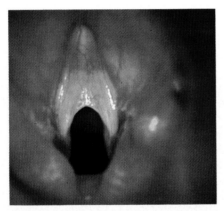

Figure 114. Larger congenital anterior glottic web in a 12-year-old with a weak, "squeaky" voice all her life. Laryngofissure, excision of web, and insertion of a keel produced a reasonably good result.

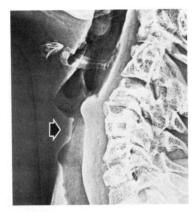

Figure 115. A large web associated with a thick subglottic stenosis (*arrow*) in a 6-year-old child with a history of a weak voice and several attacks of croup.

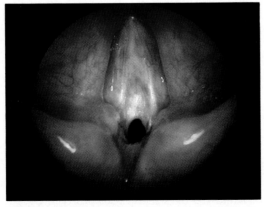

Figure 116. Endoscopic view in the same patient as in Figure 115. The outline of the vocal ligaments can be seen.

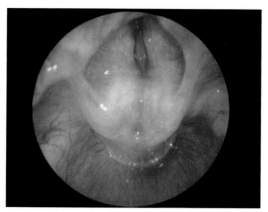

Figure 117. A baby with laryngeal atresia. At birth attempted intubation was unsuccessful and a tracheotomy was performed. There is hypoplasia of the supraglottic structures with only a rudimentary glottic outline.

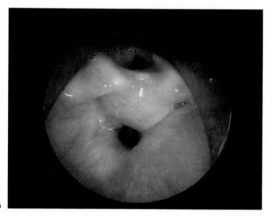

A

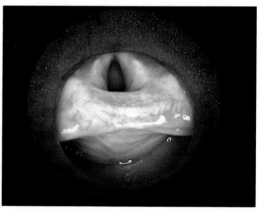

B

Figure 118. *A,* Congenital interarytenoid fixation due to a posterior glottic web. *B,* The laryngoscope is used to splay and separate the posterior commissure, and the web is stretched and clearly seen.

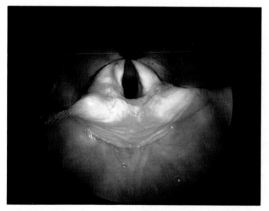

A

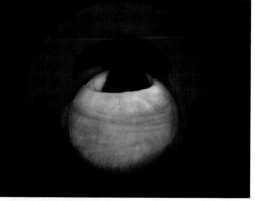

B

Figure 119. *A,* Congenital interarytenoid fixation with posterior glottic web. *B,* As in Figure 118, when a pediatric Holinger laryngoscope is used to separate the arytenoids, the web is seen.

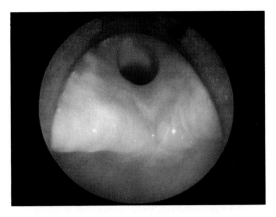

Figure 120. Posterior glottic web confined mostly to the glottic level. The web prevents vocal cord abduction and causes persistent laryngeal airway obstruction.

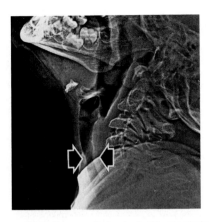

Figure 121. Congenital subglottic stenosis with a narrow airway at the cricoid level. Note that extension of the neck makes the cricoid appear to be a long way from the glottic level.

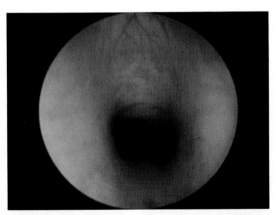

Figure 122. Subglottic stenosis in a 3-year-old. The subglottic diameter was measured as 4.5 mm.

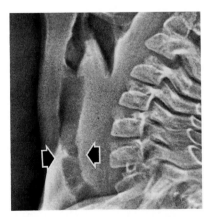

Figure 123. Lateral xerogram showing multiple congenital tracheal webs (*arrows*).

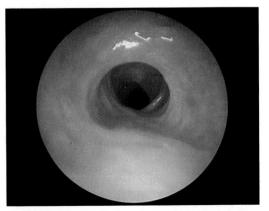

Figure 124. Endoscopy in the same case as in Figure 123 shows the congenital tracheal webs.

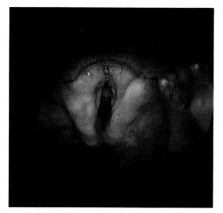

Figure 125. Posterior congenital laryngeal cleft in a patient with Opitz-Frias syndrome.

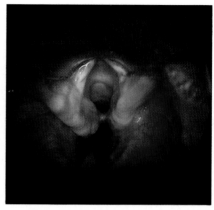

Figure 126. The same case as in Figure 125, with the blade of the laryngoscope separating the two sides of the larynx to show the posterior laryngeal cleft, which extends a few millimeters below the posterior commissure.

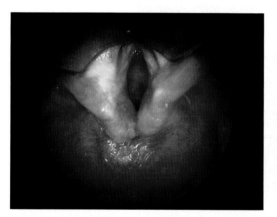

Figure 127. Posterior congenital laryngeal cleft where the cleft cannot be identified unless the laryngoscope is introduced further.

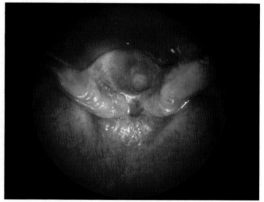

Figure 128. The laryngoscope blade separates the posterior glottis and the cleft is clearly seen.

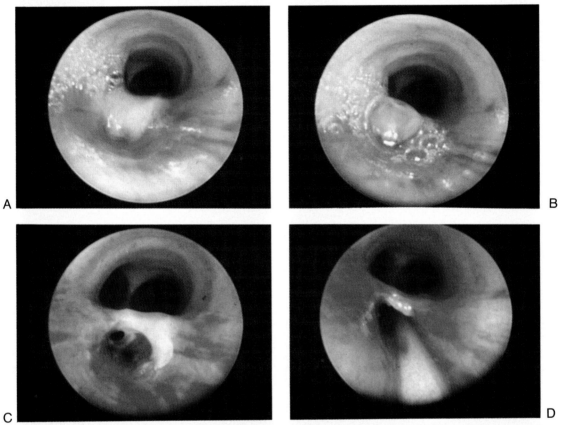

A   B

C   D

Figure 129. *A*, Esophageal atresia and lower pouch tracheoesophageal fistula in a newborn baby, 4 hours old. Endoscopic examination before repair (*B*) shows gastric juice bubbling up the fistula, and (*C*) after suction the opening of the fistula can be seen in the posterior tracheal wall. *D*, A fine catheter has been placed through the fistula to assist the surgeon at thoracotomy.

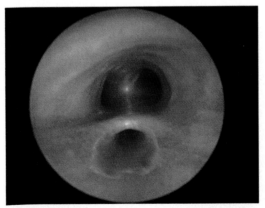

Figure 130. Lower-pouch tracheoesophageal fistula in a newborn baby. Preoperative endoscopic evaluation shows the fistula in the posterior wall of the lower trachea.

97

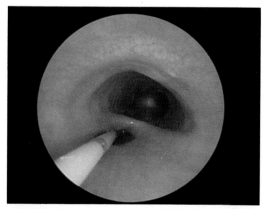

Figure 131. Tracheal aspect of a lower-pouch tracheoesophageal fistula that has not been corrected surgically. The tracheal orifice lies to the left of the midline, and a fine catheter has been passed through it.

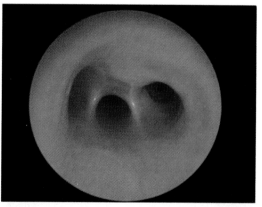

Figure 132. Opening of a tracheoesophageal fistula at the carina between the right main bronchus and the left main bronchus.

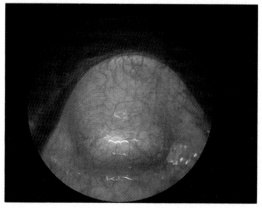

Figure 133. The blind upper esophageal pouch of esophageal atresia.

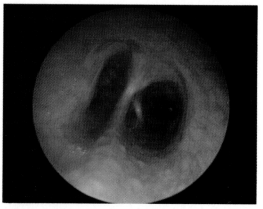

Figure 134. Bronchoesophageal fistula on the medial aspect of the right main bronchus. The orifice of the left main bronchus is elongated and of abnormal shape.

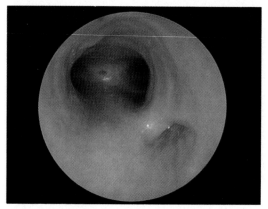

Figure 135. Blind, slitlike opening on the right posterolateral wall of the trachea. It did not lead to a tracheal bronchus, a tracheoesophageal fistula, or a sequestrated lobe.

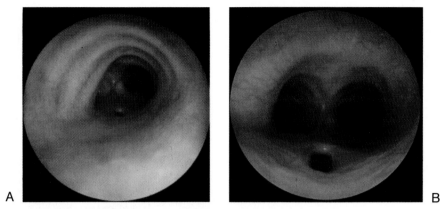

Figure 136. Small blind sinus on the posterior membranous tracheal wall just above the carina. The wide posterior membranous wall and the C-shaped tracheal cartilages (A) indicate the presence of tracheomalacia. There was no tracheoesophageal fistula or esophageal atresia. B, Close-up view.

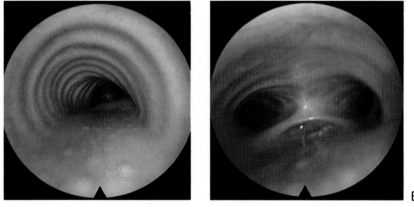

Figure 137. Trachea after operative repair of a tracheoesophageal fistula. A, The wide posterior membranous wall and C-shaped cartilages indicate tracheomalacia. B, The wide mouth of the residual pouch of the fistula is visible just above the carina, with a small blue suture showing.

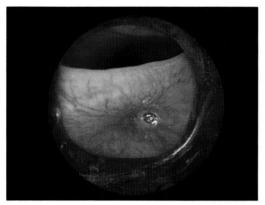

Figure 138. A bronchoscope has been introduced into the residual pouch for a few millimeters.

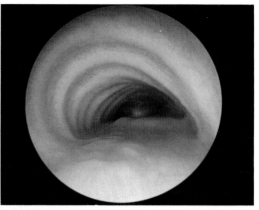

Figure 139. Tracheal aspect of repaired tracheoesophageal fistula, showing the associated changes of tracheomalacia.

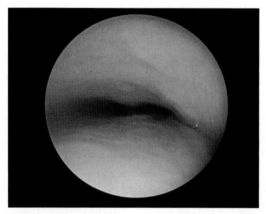

Figure 140. Severe tracheomalacia associated with tracheoesophageal fistula and esophageal atresia in a newborn baby.

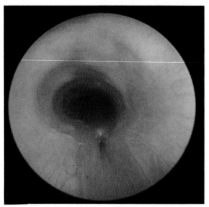

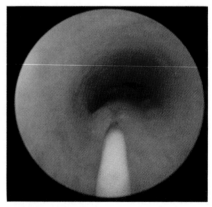

A   B

Figure 141. H-type tracheoesophageal fistula, tracheal aspect. The tracheal opening can be elusive and is seen on the posterior wall of the upper trachea (A). A fine catheter has been passed (B) to help identify the fistula at surgical division.

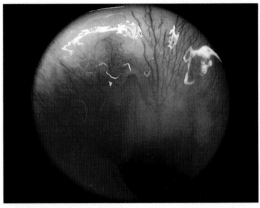

Figure 142. Esophageal aspect of an H-type tracheoesophageal fistula. This usually appears as an inverted V-shaped opening on the anterior wall of the upper esophagus, seen best as the wall is stretched with the esophagoscope and inspected with an angled telescope.

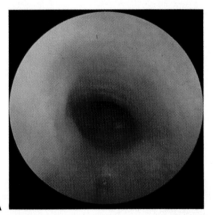

A

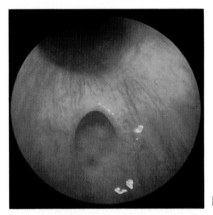

B

Figure 143. Tracheal opening of an upper-pouch fistula (A), also seen in close-up (B). In this patient the orifice is larger than usual.

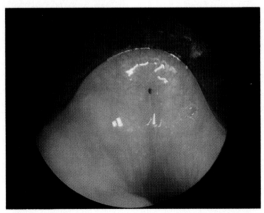

Figure 144. The tiny aperture of the esophageal aspect of an upper-pouch fistula can be very difficult to identify.

VASCULAR COMPRESSION OF THE TRACHEA, TRACHEOMALACIA, AND CONGENITAL TRACHEAL STENOSIS

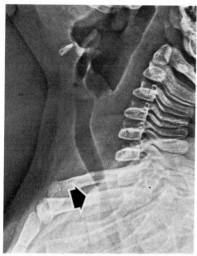

Figure 145. Mild innominate artery compression narrowing the tracheal air column (*arrow*) where the innominate artery crosses the anterior wall of the trachea in an 8-month-old baby with a barking cough, "bronchitis," and retained secretions.

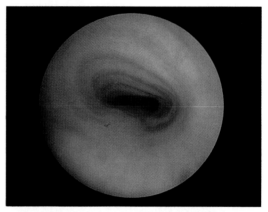

Figure 146. Tracheal compression by the innominate artery at the junction of the upper two thirds and lower third of the trachea. The ratio of the width of the posterior membranous wall to the internal perimeter of the tracheal cartilages is the normal 1 to 4.5.

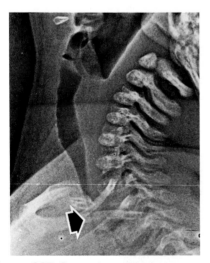

Figure 147. Severe innominate artery compression with marked narrowing (*arrow*) of the lower third of the trachea.

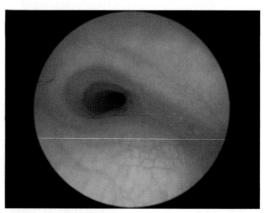

Figure 148. Severe innominate artery compression, with the right anterior and posterior walls of the trachea touching one another. The posterior membranous wall is wide and balloons forward. The ratio of membranous wall to tracheal cartilage is 1 to 2.

102

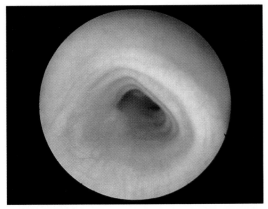

Figure 149. Double aortic arch. The narrowed tracheal aspect shows an almost triangular appearance.

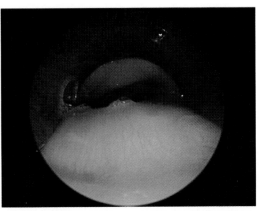

Figure 150. The posterior arch of a double aortic arch passing behind the esophagus at the junction of the upper third and the lower two thirds.

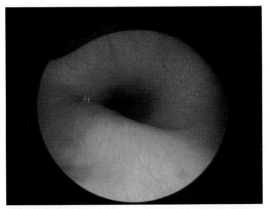

Figure 151. Annomalous right subclavian artery that causes no symptoms passing behind the upper esophagus. This appearance must be differentiated from the posterior arch of a double aortic arch.

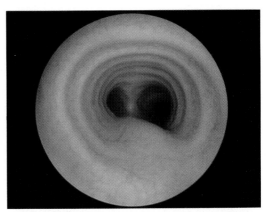

Figure 152. Right subclavian artery that passes behind the esophagus is seen through the posterior membranous tracheal wall as a pulsatile bulge.

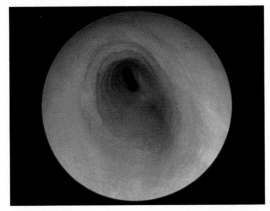

Figure 153. Vascular compression of the right anterolateral wall of the upper trachea by a right common carotid artery that arose from a common trunk.

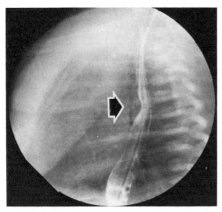

Figure 154. Vascular sling seen on a lateral x-ray during barium swallow. The left pulmonary artery occupies the space between the trachea and the esophagus (*arrow*).

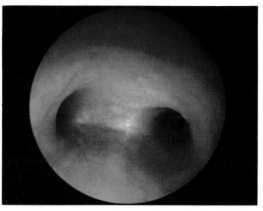

Figure 155. Endoscopic view of a vascular sling seen as a compressible fullness behind the posterior wall of the lower trachea.

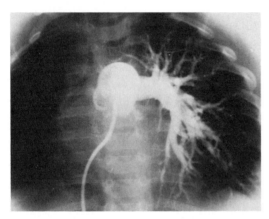

Figure 156. A huge single pulmonary artery seen at angiography.

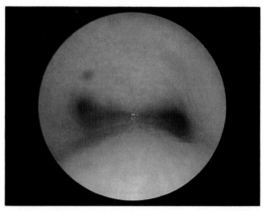

Figure 157. Compression of the carina and the orifices of the left and right main bronchus by a large pulmonary artery.

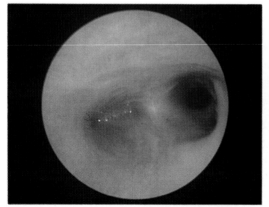

Figure 158. The left main bronchus is seen to be almost totally obstructed by a dilated, hypertensive pulmonary artery.

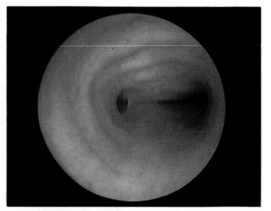

Figure 159. Compression of the lower trachea and carina in a patient with tetralogy of Fallot.

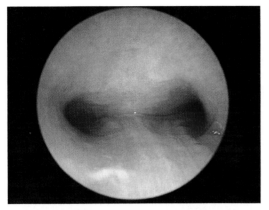

Figure 160. Compression of the lower trachea and carina by a paratracheal mediastinal hemangioma.

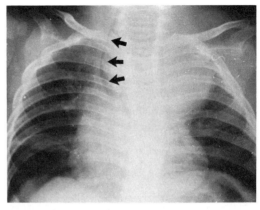

Figure 161. Compression of the intrathoracic trachea by a mediastinal lymphosarcoma (*arrows*).

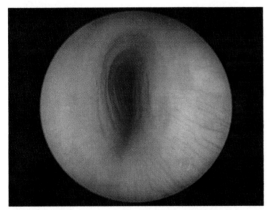

Figure 162. Side-to-side compression of the lower trachea by a neuroblastoma in a 1-month-old baby.

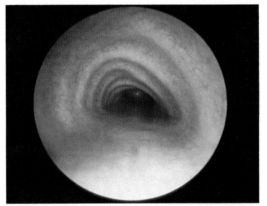

Figure 163. Primary tracheomalacia. The lower trachea shows the typical changes of narrowed lumen, widened posterior membranous wall, and C-shaped indented tracheal cartilages with a membranous wall to cartilage ratio 1 to 2.

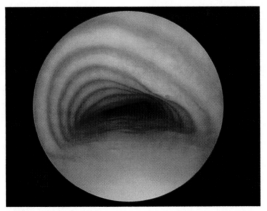

Figure 164. Another case of tracheomalacia with severe narrowing of the lumen.

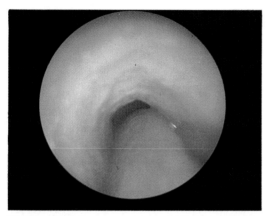

Figure 165. Severe tracheomalacia in a 2-week-old infant, associated with tracheoesophageal fistula that has been repaired. There is forward ballooning of the widened posterior membranous wall.

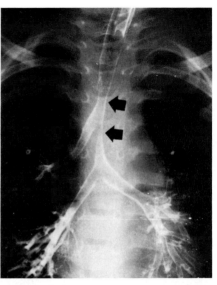

Figure 166. Severe congenital stenosis of the lower trachea both above and below a right-sided tracheal bronchus (*arrows*). No associated vascular sling was ever demonstrated.

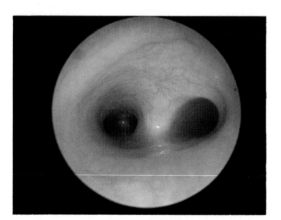

Figure 167. The orifice of a right tracheal bronchus is on the right, and the very narrowed lower tracheal lumen is on the left.

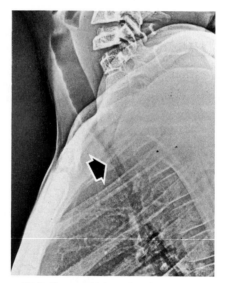

Figure 168. Congenital tracheal stenosis. Lateral xerogram showing a normal upper trachea and a uniformly narrowed lower trachea (*arrow*).

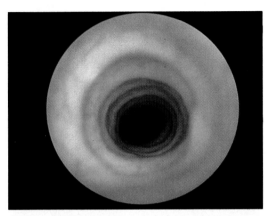

Figure 169. Complete rigid cartilaginous rings, typical of congenital tracheal stenosis.

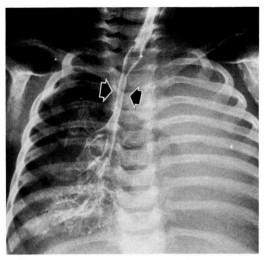

Figure 170. Tracheobronchogram showing aplasia of the left lung and stenosis (*arrows*) of the airway leading to the only functional lung tissue on the right.

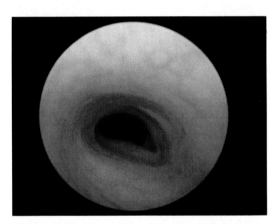

Figure 171. The endoscopic view shows congenital stenosis of the trachea, which was not distensible for passage of even the smallest bronchoscope.

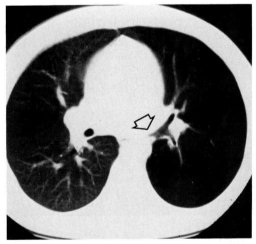

Figure 172. Bronchogenic cyst. CT shows overdistention of left lung caused by compression of the left main bronchus (*arrow*).

ACUTE INFLAMMATORY AIRWAY OBSTRUCTION

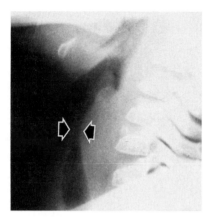

Figure 173. Acute laryngotracheitis (croup) with narrowing of the subglottic airway (*arrows*) by edema. In other examples the x-ray may show diffuse haziness in the subglottic region.

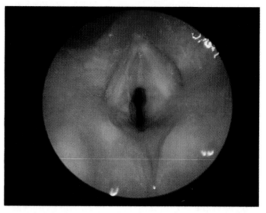

Figure 174. Acute laryngotracheitis with severe inflammation and subglottic edema photographed before intubation for airway obstruction.

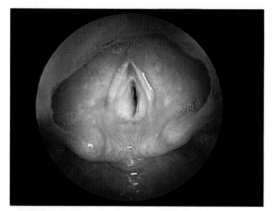

Figure 175. Another example of severe laryngotracheitis. The vocal cords are clearly seen and there is no abnormality of the supraglottic structures.

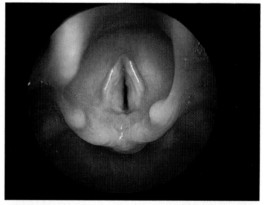

Figure 176. Acute laryngotracheitis with severe subglottic inflammation and swelling.

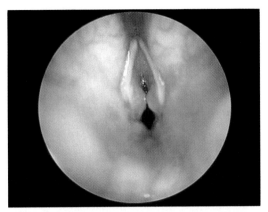

Figure 177. Persistent subglottic edema in acute laryngotracheitis treated by endotracheal intubation. Extubation failed at 8 days and a tracheotomy was performed.

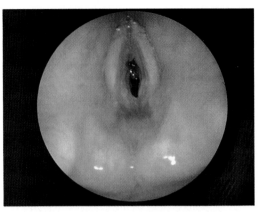

Figure 178. Acute pseudomembranous croup, a severe form of acute laryngotracheitis in a child with a toxic reaction and a high fever. *Staphylococcus aureus* was isolated from tracheal culture.

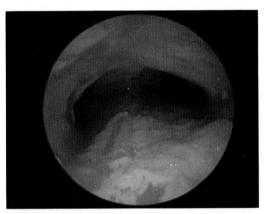

Figure 179. The ulcerated surface of the trachea in pseudomembranous croup, after crusts had been removed at bronchoscopy.

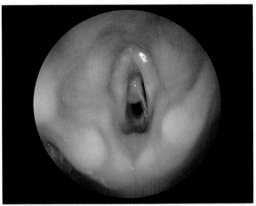

Figure 180. Impacted subglottic foreign body with surrounding granulations, giving clinical features of prolonged croup.

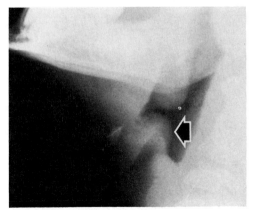

Figure 181. Acute epiglottitis with gross swelling of the epiglottis (*arrow*). Care must be taken that positioning for the x-ray does not make the respiratory obstruction worse. X-ray is usually not necessary.

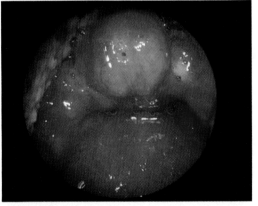

Figure 182. Acute epiglottitis and some swelling of the surrounding tissues. There is a very narrow, pinpoint airway.

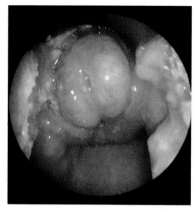
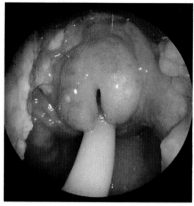

A

B

Figure 183. Acute epiglottitis (*A*) before intubation and (*B*) after intubation.

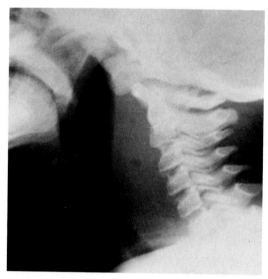

Figure 184. Acute retropharyngeal abscess on a lateral x-ray. The infant presented with high fever, toxicity, and upper airway obstruction.

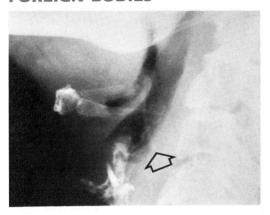

Figure 185. An adult with a fishbone (*arrow*) behind the epiglottis.

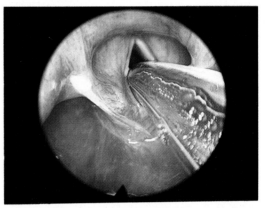

Figure 186. Same patient as in Figure 185. The fishbone is embedded, lying parallel to the left aryepiglottic fold.

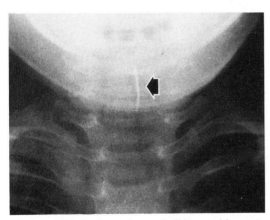

Figure 187. A piece of egg shell (*arrow*) impacted in the glottic opening in a baby.

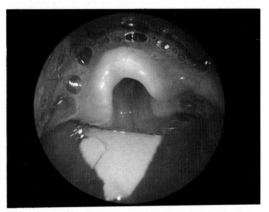

Figure 188. Same patient as in Figure 187. The egg shell has been carefully manipulated from the glottic opening, which was inflamed and edematous. The egg shell has fallen on the posterior pharyngeal wall prior to final removal.

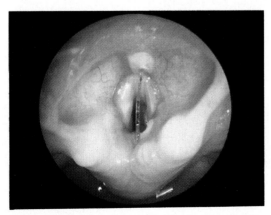

Figure 189. Glass fragment of a broken electric light bulb, inhaled and impacted in the glottic opening in an 8-month-old baby.

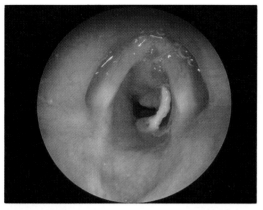

Figure 190. Granulation tissue surrounding a piece of bone that was impacted in the subglottic region of a child for many days.

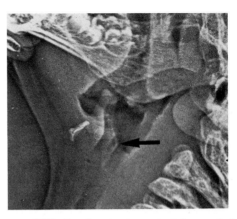

Figure 191. Foreign body, a leaf (*arrow*), inhaled and embedded in the supraglottic larynx.

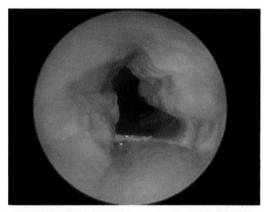

Figure 192. Endoscopic appearance of a piece of apple core inhaled into the upper trachea 10 weeks before endoscopic removal. Marked inflammatory change and granulation tissue reaction at the site of impaction.

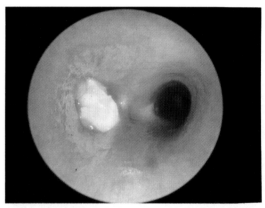

Figure 193. Fragment of a nut inhaled into the left main bronchus.

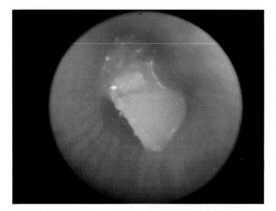

Figure 194. A peanut fragment in the right main bronchus prior to endoscopic removal.

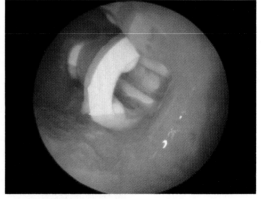

Figure 195. Plastic foreign body in the right main bronchus. Most plastic foreign bodies are not radiopaque.

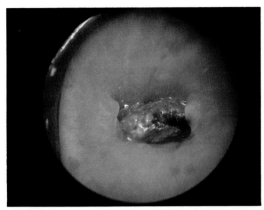

Figure 196. A stone impacted in the right main bronchus.

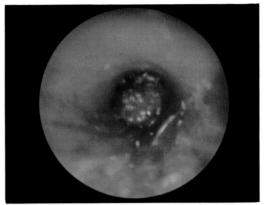

Figure 197. Dry secretions impacted in the trachea of an infant being ventilated via an endotracheal tube. Bronchoscopy is essential to remove such discrete, dry obstructions.

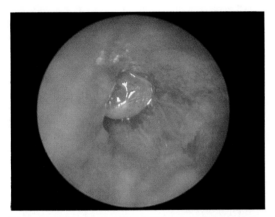

Figure 198. Granulation tissue almost completely obstructing the right main bronchus after a foreign body has been removed.

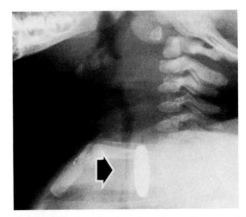

Figure 199. A coin that has been impacted in the esophagus for 6 days. Surrounding inflammatory swelling has caused narrowing of the tracheal air column (*arrow*).

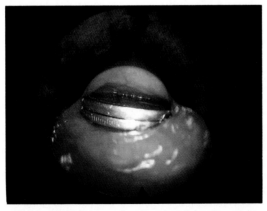

Figure 200. Two coins impacted in the upper esophagus.

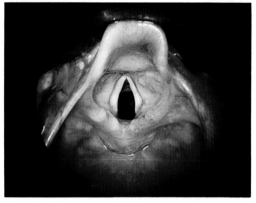

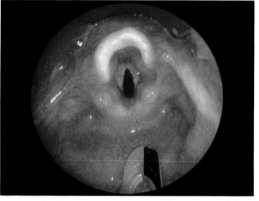

Figure 201. A child's normal laryngopharynx exposed with a Lindholm laryngoscope and the child under general anesthesia with spontaneous respiration.

Figure 202. A pernasal pharyngeal tube insufflates oxygen in an infant at the end of diagnostic endoscopy, when the dynamics of the larynx can be evaluated. No perlaryngeal endotracheal tube is used during diagnostic endoscopy.

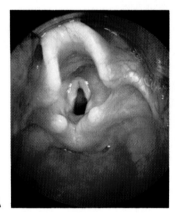

A

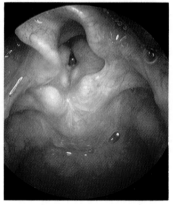

B

Figure 203. Laryngeal spasm. *A,* The normal larynx in an infant under spontaneous respiration anesthesia. *B,* Temporary laryngeal spasm.

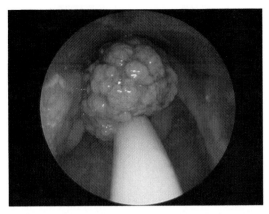

Figure 204. An adolescent patient with a large mass of papilloma in the supraglottic region causing partial airway obstruction. An endotracheal tube is passed temporarily to relieve the obstruction, deepen the anesthesia, and allow removal of the mass.

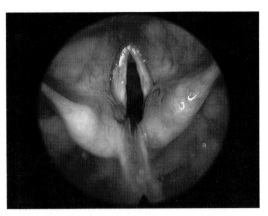

Figure 205. Normal adult larynx under general anesthesia with a relaxant technique and jet ventilation using the Benjamin jet anesthesia tube (2.8 mm external diameter).

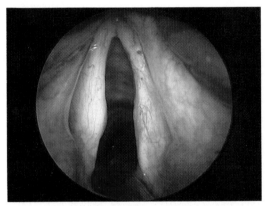

Figure 206. An adult patient with a paralyzed left vocal cord just prior to injection of Teflon. The jet anesthesia tube lies unobtrusively in the posterior commissure.

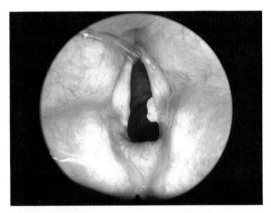

Figure 207. The jet tube for anesthesia has been manipulated into the anterior commissure so that a vocal granuloma can be removed.

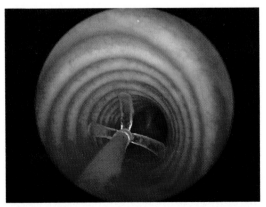

Figure 208. The distal tip of the jet tube in the mid-trachea. The four soft plastic petals maintain it in position.

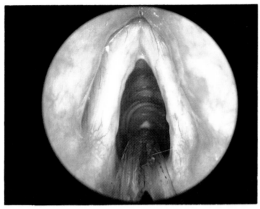

Figure 209. A 5 mm internal diameter microlaryngoscopy endotracheal tube in an adult, lying in the posterior commissure and partly obscuring it. The cuff of the endotracheal tube can be seen inflated in the trachea. The patient is paralyzed and ventilated.

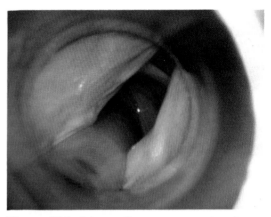

Figure 210. A large-diameter armored endotracheal tube lying in the posterior commissure of an adult larynx that has bilateral vocal ulcers. The pathology can be seen, but the endotracheal tube obscures the posterior commissure.

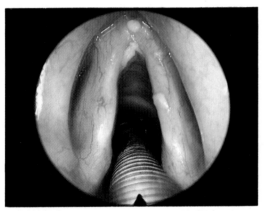

Figure 211. A Laser-Flex tube for general anesthesia and safer laser surgery in the larynx. In this patient, visualization of anterior pathology is excellent.

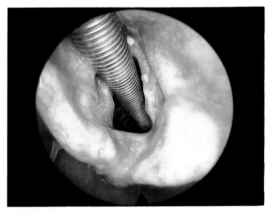

Figure 212. The Laser-Flex tube is too large and awkward to be easily manipulated into the anterior larynx.

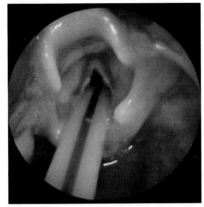
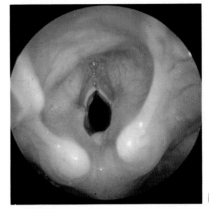

A   B

Figure 213. Ulceration in a neonate intubated for 5 days. *A,* With the tube in situ, there is ulceration of the edge of both vocal cords in the region of the vocal process. *B,* After the tube has been removed, the ulceration is seen more clearly. These changes usually resolve within 7 to 10 days.

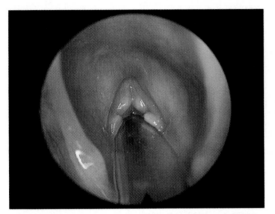
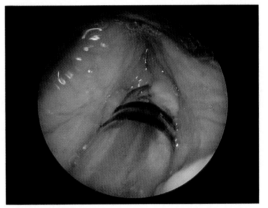

Figure 214. Granulation tissue forming at each vocal process. The anterior part of the vocal folds is edematous.

Figure 215. A close-up shows granulation tissue from each vocal process on the anterior surface of the tube.

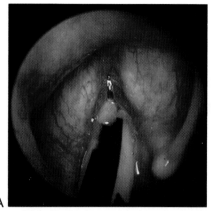
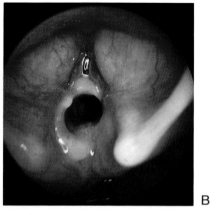

A

B

Figure 216. *A,* With the tube in the larynx, a true appreciation of the laryngeal trauma cannot be obtained. *B,* The extent of the damage is revealed when the tube is removed.

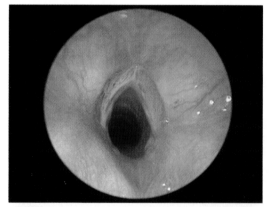
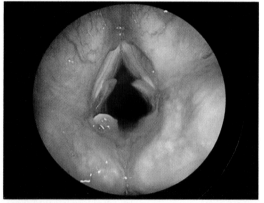

Figure 217. Minimal swelling and congestion with mild mucosal reaction in a neonate intubated for 9 days.

Figure 218. Granulation tissue arising from the medial surface of the arytenoids and in the posterior commissure on the left side.

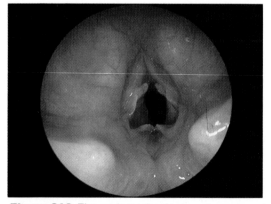

Figure 219. The endotracheal tube was removed immediately before this photograph, which shows granulation tissue that had formed around the tube.

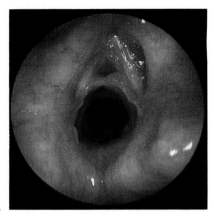
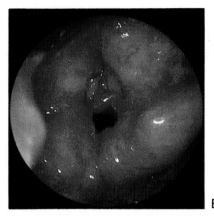

A

B

Figure 220. A, Marked mucosal reaction and fresh granulation tissue from the vocal process after extubation. B, Some minutes later, the soft tissues are more swollen. The airway is reduced, there is gross distortion of the larynx, and the reason for failure to successfully extubate is obvious.

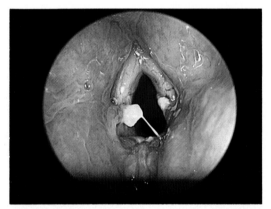

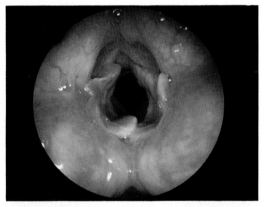

Figure 221. Yellow color in the vocal cords reflecting generalized jaundice in a woman who was intubated for 10 days for liver failure.

Figure 222. Severe intubation trauma with abundant granulation tissue. Ulceration in the subglottic region can be suspected.

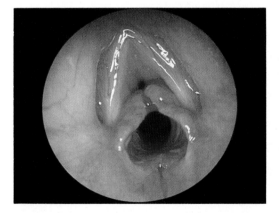

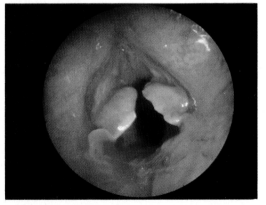

Figure 223. Large "flaps" of granulation tissue which, as they swell, will cause a ball-valve obstruction in the larynx.

Figure 224. The granulation tissue "flaps" move in and out with respiration.

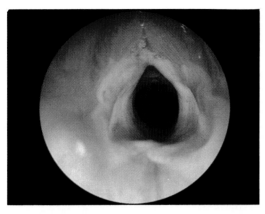

Figure 225. Granulation tissue in the posterior glottis. In the subglottic space there is ulceration through the perichondrium circumferentially into cartilage. Fibrous tissue may later form an annular, firm subglottic stenosis.

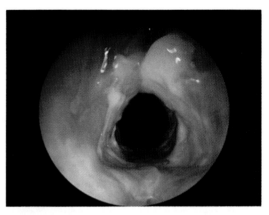

Figure 226. Extensive, advanced intubation trauma with ulceration seen to be going into cartilage and the cricoarytenoid joints and forming bilateral ulcerated "troughs."

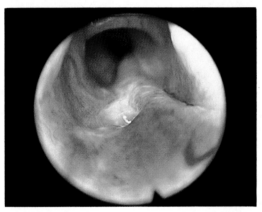

Figure 227. An unusual case with necrosis of the posterior surface of the cricoid cartilage forming a chronic fistula between the subglottic region and the upper esophagus. The opening of the fistula can be seen.

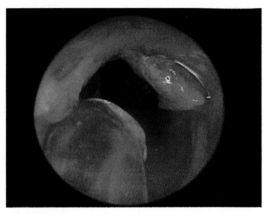

Figure 228. A large piece of granulation tissue in the lower trachea at the site of constant friction from the tip of an endotracheal tube.

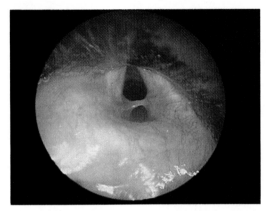

Figure 229. Delicate interarytenoid adhesion that formed after 2 weeks of intubation in a small baby.

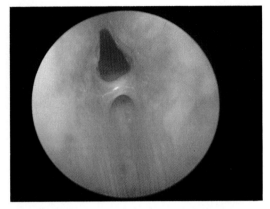

Figure 230. A thick band of tissue in the subglottic region with a triangular aperture in front and a circular aperture behind.

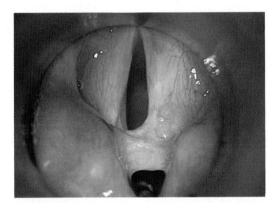

Figure 231. "Bilateral vocal cord paralysis" was diagnosed. In fact, the fibrous band between the vocal cords made abduction impossible.

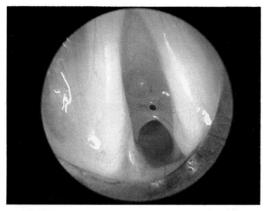

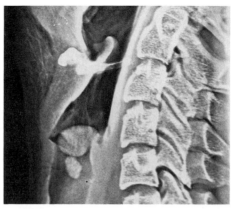

Figure 232. Obstructing subglottic membranous web with a tiny hole in the posterior part of the membrane.

Figure 233. Intubation granulomas that formed following 5 days of intubation after bilateral mandibular osteotomies in a young woman. There was serious airway obstruction necessitating a tracheotomy using local anesthesia.

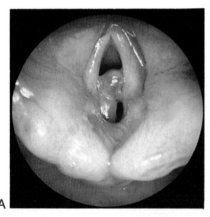

A

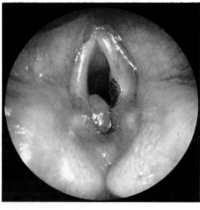

B

Figure 234. *A,* Bilateral intubation granulomas following intubation for airway burns. *B,* One granuloma has been removed with the laser.

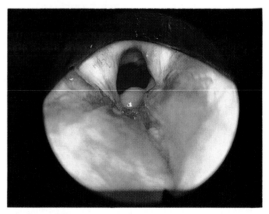

Figure 235. Granuloma at the anterior end of the left vocal cord that formed after intubation for removal of the gall bladder. The intubation was difficult, and an introducer was used in the endotracheal tube. Intubation trauma was probably the basis of chronic granuloma formation.

Figure 236. Rounded granulation with surrounding edema and congestion following intubation for 2 weeks in a paraplegic woman.

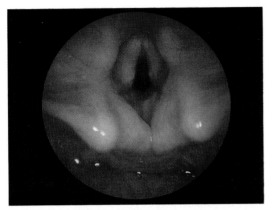

Figure 237. Granulation tissue, which is maturing to fibrous tissue, filling the posterior glottis and beginning to form a scar.

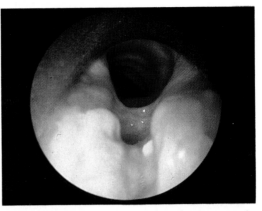

Figure 238. Mature posterior glottic stenosis. There is a web at the glottic level and interarytenoid fibrosis that limits vocal cord abduction.

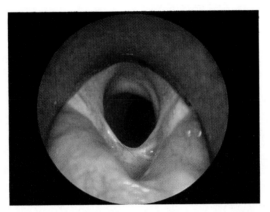

Figure 239. Posterior glottic web and interarytenoid fibrosis clearly demonstrated by separating and splaying the vocal cords with a laryngoscope.

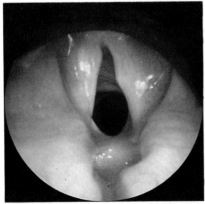

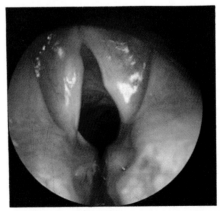

Figure 240. *A*, Mature posterior glottic stenosis causing moderate airway obstruction. *B*, The transverse fibrotic scar has been divided with a curved scalpel blade on a long handle. The tissues have parted, leaving a deep V-shaped defect where the stenosis is "released."

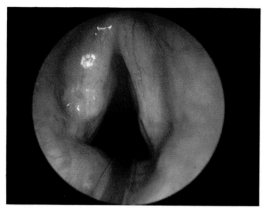

Figure 241. Chronic intubation trauma with irregular edema of the left vocal fold and a scarred healed "furrow" where an acute ulcerated "trough" had been caused by the indwelling tube. It is reasonable to assume that the cricoarytenoid joint is affected.

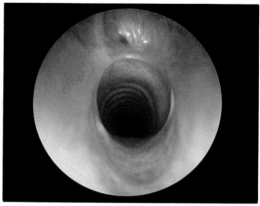

Figure 242. Subglottic web, mostly anterior, seen with the 30° telescope.

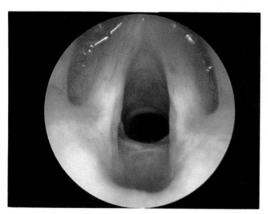

Figure 243. Subglottic stenosis, mostly posterior.

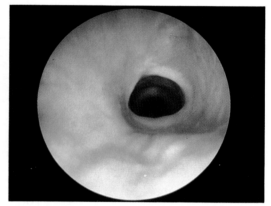

Figure 244. Mature subglottic stenosis narrowing the airway.

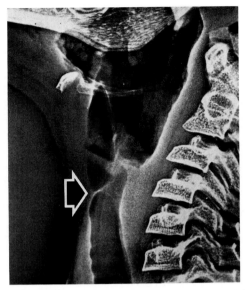

Figure 245. Lateral xerogram showing a thin subglottic web (*arrow*).

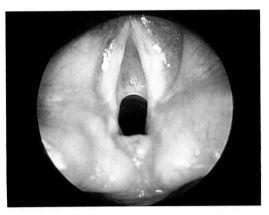

Figure 246. The subglottic web is mostly anterior. It responded to laser treatment and a normal airway was achieved.

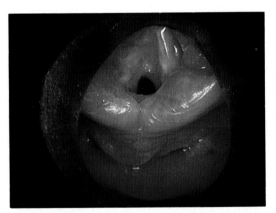

Figure 247. Chronic changes following trauma from prolonged intubation. The left vocal cord is almost unrecognizable in scar tissue, and there is severe stenosis of the glottic and subglottic region.

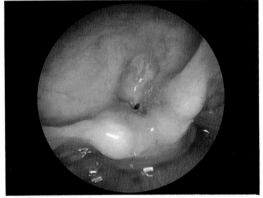

Figure 248. Chronic laryngeal stenosis with distortion and rotation of the larynx following prolonged intubation in an adolescent child with a head injury.

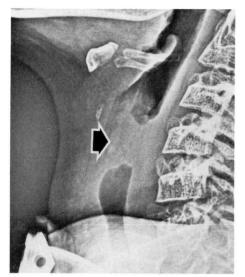

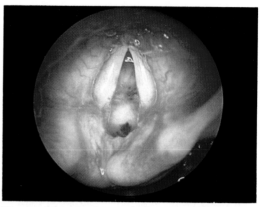

Figure 249. Total obstruction in the glottic and subglottic region following endotracheal tube trauma for which a tracheotomy was performed. The x-ray shows the thickness (*arrow*) of the obstruction.

Figure 250. The same patient as in Figure 249, at endoscopy. A laryngoplasty restored a reasonably good airway, and the tracheotomy was removed.

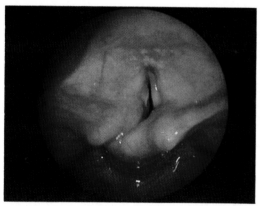

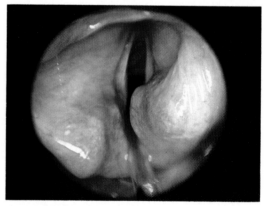

Figure 251. Dislocation of the left arytenoid with fixation of the left vocal cord. An erroneous diagnosis of left vocal cord paralysis had been made. Endoscopic arytenoidectomy restored a good airway, and the tracheotomy tube, which had been present for 3 years, was removed within 10 days.

Figure 252. Adult patient with dislocation of the right arytenoid caused by intubation for general anesthesia.

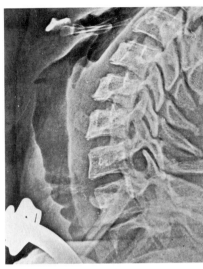

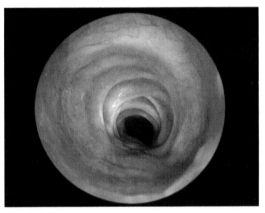

Figure 253. Multiple concentric annular fibrous strictures of the trachea that formed at the site of the inflated cuff of an endotracheal tube left in situ for 2 weeks following a head injury.

Figure 254. Same patient as in Figure 253. The stenoses are seen at several levels in the trachea.

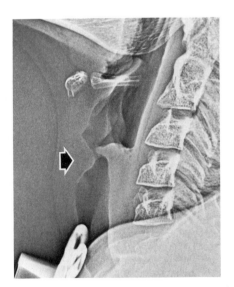

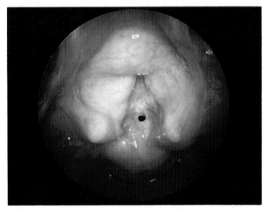

Figure 255. Severe chronic stenosis at the glottic level both anterior and posterior, with only a small airway (*arrow*).

Figure 256. Same patient as in Figure 255. At endoscopy the airway is about 2 mm and the severe supraglottic and glottic webbing can be seen.

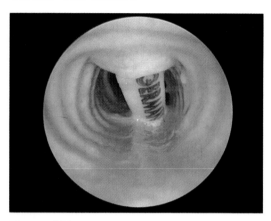

Figure 257. An endotracheal anesthesia tube passed through the tracheostome into the lower trachea.

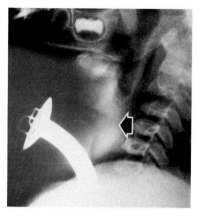

Figure 258. A high tracheotomy (*arrow*) has been repositioned. The best site for a tracheotomy in a pediatric patient is the third and fourth tracheal cartilages.

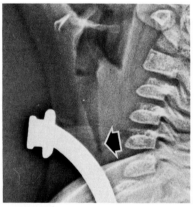

Figure 259. There is a tracheal "flap," a localized area of tracheomalacia due to pressure of the tracheotomy tube on the anterior wall of the trachea, just above the tracheostoma (*arrow*).

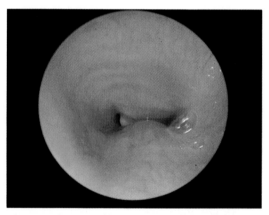

Figure 260. Endoscopic photograph confirming the presence of "tracheal flap" above the internal site of the tracheostome.

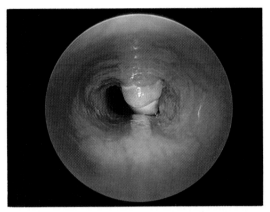

Figure 261. Granulations at the inner aspect of a tracheotomy site form often and are usually easy to remove before decannulation.

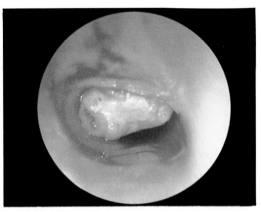

Figure 262. These granulations at the tracheotomy site were unusual, as they became very firm and were difficult to remove.

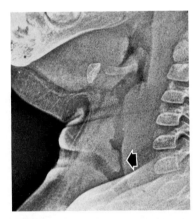

Figure 263. Granulations at the tracheotomy site (*arrow*) on the lateral xerogram, which has been taken with the tracheotomy tube removed.

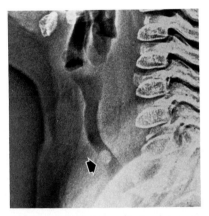

Figure 264. Rounded granulation at the tracheotomy site (*arrow*) in a patient whose tracheotomy tube had been removed about 10 weeks before. This complication is rare.

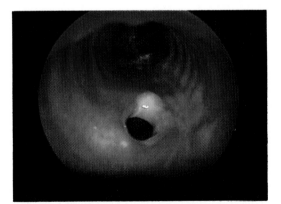

Figure 265. Large traumatic perforation of the posterior membranous wall of the trachea in an adult woman. A soft Silastic tracheotomy tube with a hard plastic introducer was the cause of this complication.

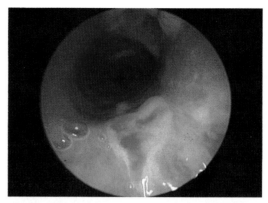

Figure 266. The posterior membranous tracheal wall in a child who had a tracheotomy 2 weeks before. The tracheotomy tube is causing ulceration on the posterior wall, and a smaller tube is needed.

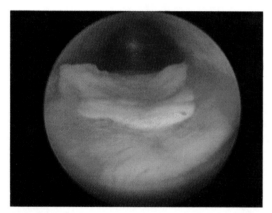

Figure 267. Large area of ulceration on the posterior tracheal wall caused by a tracheotomy tube in a premature baby.

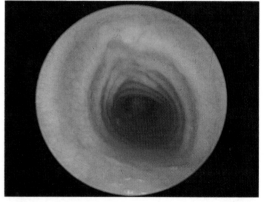

Figure 268. Scar of a previous tracheotomy on the anterior wall of the upper trachea. The scar is typically a small dimple.

LARYNGEAL TRAUMA

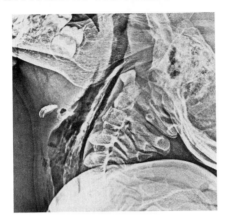

Figure 269. Surgical emphysema in the prevertebral and neck tissues after traumatic rupture of the tracheoesophageal wall. A 3-year-old fell, striking the front of his neck on a blunt object. The skin remained intact, but the posterior tracheal wall ruptured. Healing was uneventful with no operation.

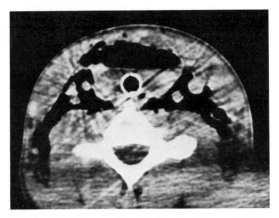

Figure 270. Severe blunt injury to the trachea in a young woman causing complete distraction of the cricoid cartilage from the upper trachea. The endotracheal tube is lying in a space containing blood and air with extensive surgical emphysema in the lateral neck on both sides.

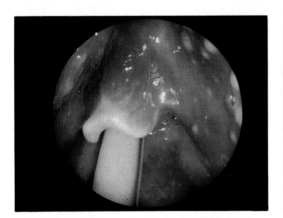

Figure 271. Submucosal hemorrhage in the vallecula in a boy hit on the neck while playing football. There was no fracture or dislocation of the laryngeal framework, and healing was uneventful.

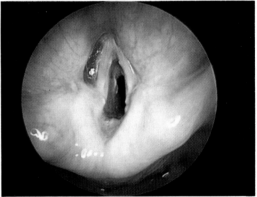

Figure 272. Submucosal hematoma in the left ventricle and in the subglottic region in a patient who fell and struck her neck on the edge of a bathtub.

131

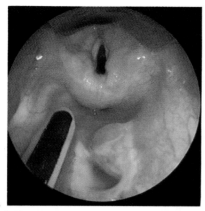
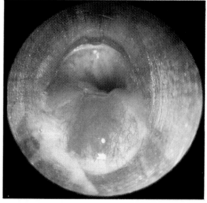

A

B

Figure 273. "Unsuccessful" endotracheal intubation was followed by bleeding in a newborn baby. *A,* The large traumatic laceration on the posterior wall of the pharynx was caused by misdirection of the endotracheal tube behind the larynx into the prevertebral space and the mediastinum. *B,* Hematoma behind the posterior wall of the mid-esophagus.

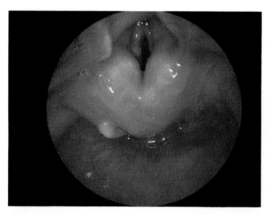
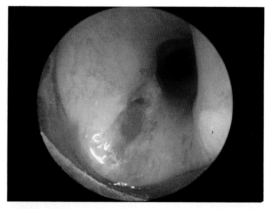

Figure 274. Ulceration of the posterior surface of the left arytenoid caused by nasogastric intubation for 10 days.

Figure 275. Penetrating dog bite injury in the upper trachea. The patient was savaged by a dog, had over 40 bite marks, and required more than 100 sutures to various lacerations.

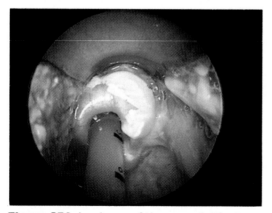
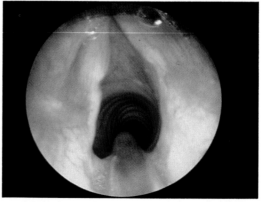

Figure 276. Lye burns of the supraglottic structures and epiglottis in a 4-year-old.

Figure 277. Defect in the left vocal cord with scarring following a previous excessively large biopsy for a benign condition. The voice was permanently affected.

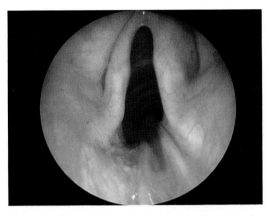

Figure 278. Small web at the anterior commissure in a woman who had vocal nodules "stripped" from both the right and left cords at the same operation. Permanent minor dysphonia resulted.

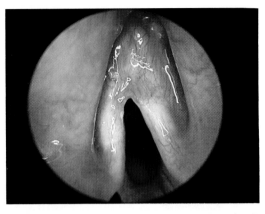

Figure 279. A moderate-sized anterior glottic adhesion in an older man who had multiple laser treatments over 7 years for recurring epithelial dysplasia and carcinoma-in-situ.

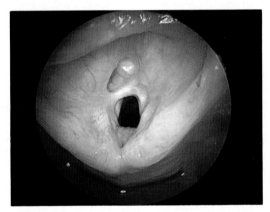

Figure 280. Severe scarring of the larynx and a firm fibrous web between the false cords following injudicious surgery for papilloma in a 15-year-old boy.

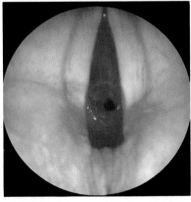
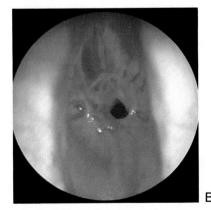

A   B

Figure 281. Severe acquired subglottic stenosis from prolonged intubation in a middle-aged woman. The vocal cords are normal (A), but there is only a small subglottic aperture (B).

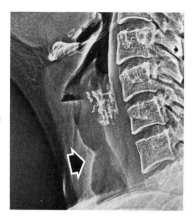

Figure 282. Subglottic stenosis, mainly anterior (*arrow*), in a 20-year-old woman. Xerogram shows that the stenosis extends over several centimeters.

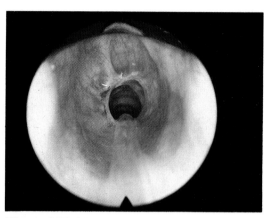

Figure 283. Idiopathic subglottic stenosis. Multiple biopsies and microbiological studies were negative.

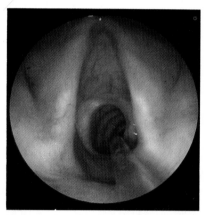

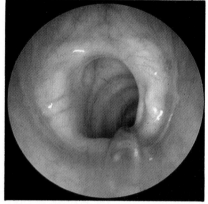

Figure 284. Normal glottis (*left*) but a mature symmetric, annular, fibrous stenosis in the subglottic region, the site of primary repair of complete rupture of the airway in a motor vehicle accident.

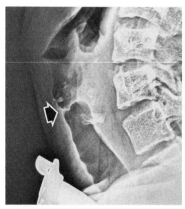

Figure 285. Thin diaphragm (*arrow*) in the subglottic region of a 7-year-old intubated for croup for 7 days. Tracheotomy for "failed extubation."

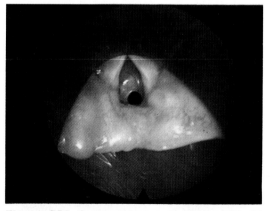

Figure 286. Same patient as in Figure 285. At endoscopy the presence of the diaphragm is confirmed, and there is a small central aperture. Two laser treatments restored a normal airway, and the tracheotomy tube was promptly removed.

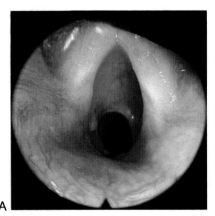 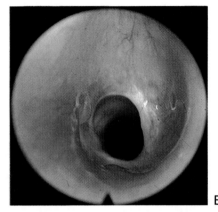

A   B

Figure 287. *A,* Subglottic stenosis following prolonged intubation for croup. No tracheotomy was performed. Laser treatment led to a good result (*B*).

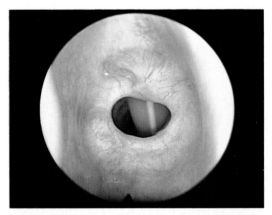 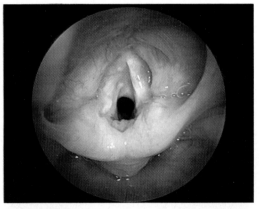

Figure 288. Close-up of a mature subglottic stenosis of about 5 mm diameter. The plastic tube through the tracheotomy below the web must be changed to a laser-proof tube and protected before laser treatment is commenced.

Figure 289. High subglottic web and fibrous scar of the left vocal cord with a fixed left cricoarytenoid joint in a 13-year-old who crushed his larynx when he fell off a bicycle.

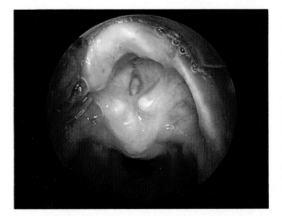 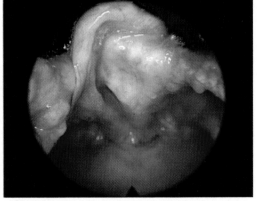

Figure 290. Complete closure of the larynx, scar tissue at the vocal cord level, and a thick posterior glottic stenosis with no subglottic stenosis. The patient originally had a partial glottic stenosis and was "treated" with over 20 laser operations until finally there was an airway fire during laser surgery. Laryngoplasty and long-term stenting were required.

Figure 291. Gross distortion, fibrosis, and complete obstruction in the larynx of a 4-year-old child who had been inappropriately treated with repeated laser operations. Laryngoplasty was required.

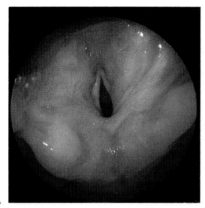
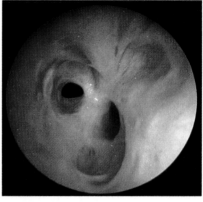

A

B

Figure 292. Scarring from airway burns in a child who had been in a locked motor vehicle and was playing with matches when the interior of the car caught fire. *A*, Severe posterior glottic stenosis *B*, Narrowing, scarring, and irregular stenosis of the trachea.

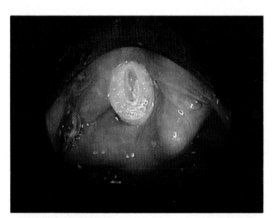

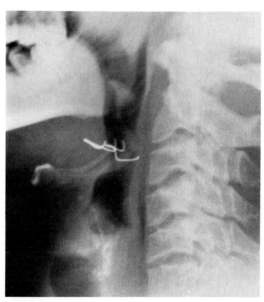

Figure 293. A firm Silastic roll in the larynx and subglottic region, which was sewn in for 4 months for the surgical treatment of subglottic stenosis.

Figure 294. Impacted dentures penetrated the pharyngeal wall in a 27-year-old mentally retarded patient. Only the wire in the dentures is radiopaque. There is surgical emphysema in the prevertebral space.

VOCAL NODULES AND CHRONIC LARYNGITIS

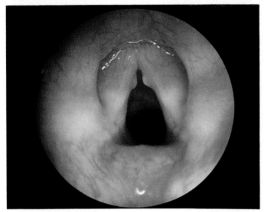

Figure 295. Prominent edematous vocal nodules in a 6-month-old child. The nodules are anterior because the membranous vocal fold at this age is the anterior half of the glottis, the vocal process being in the middle of the vocal cord.

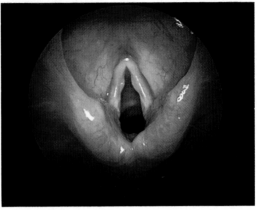

Figure 296. Symmetrical bilateral vocal nodules in a 10-year-old.

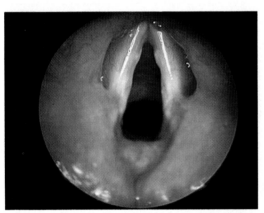

Figure 297. Vocal nodules in an adolescent. There is surface nodularity and thickening at the typical site, with surrounding edema extending into the edge of each vocal fold. Note the edema in the anterior subcommissure.

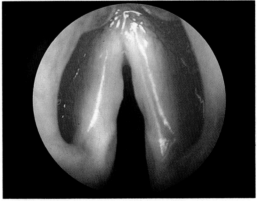

Figure 298. Vocal nodules seen with a 30° telescope, emphasizing the fusiform edematous swelling of the edge and undersurface of the vocal folds.

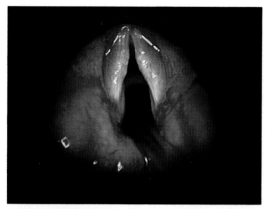

Figure 299. Hypertrophic granular vocal nodules with associated Reinke's edema in a 20-year-old female singer who had a demanding singing role in a popular musical.

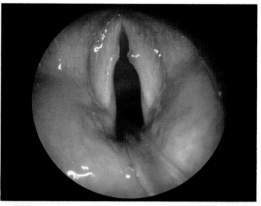

Figure 300. Vocal nodules in a young woman, with recent hemorrhage into the right nodule.

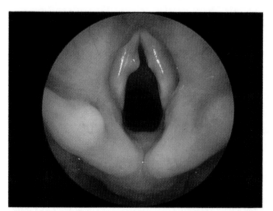

Figure 301. The left vocal nodule is larger than the corresponding nodule on the other side. This aroused a suspicion that there might be an intramucosal cyst, which was not so in this case.

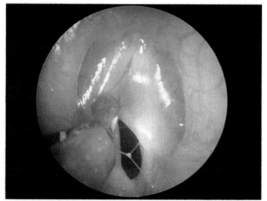

Figure 302. The right vocal nodule was grasped by a cup-shaped forceps and retracted to emphasize the longitudinal extension of edema. Curved scissors were then used to remove the focal nodularity and the area of perinodular edema.

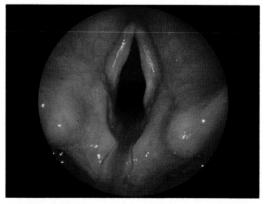

Figure 303. Chronic laryngitis in an adult with some fusiform swelling of the left vocal cord resembling a nodule, but there is no nodule on the right. There is some generalized edema in Reinke's space in both vocal cords.

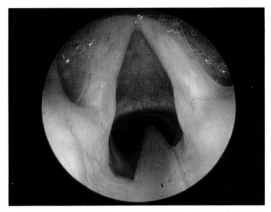

Figure 304. The left vocal cord is different from the right in a woman with persistent dysphonia. A laryngeal operation had been done previously, and submucosal scarring is probably the cause of her dysphonia.

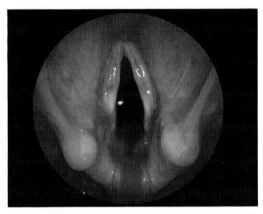

Figure 305. Chronic laryngitis in a patient with proven Hashimoto's disease.

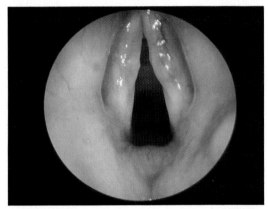

Figure 306. Subepithelial inclusion cysts were seen in the biopsy specimen from the larynx of a 4-year-old boy with a persistently husky voice. Both vocal folds have an irregular surface and edge.

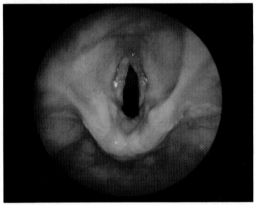

Figure 307. Chronic laryngitis in an adult with a persistently husky voice. Findings on biopsy were nonspecific, and no cause was identified.

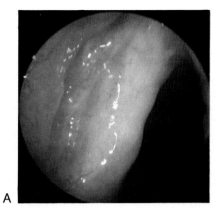
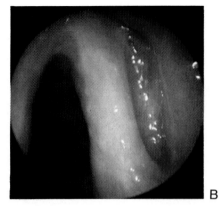

A

B

Figure 308. Chronic laryngitis. Close-up view of the vocal folds on both the left side (A) and the right side (B) with a 30° telescope, showing irregular thickening of the surface and in Reinke's space.

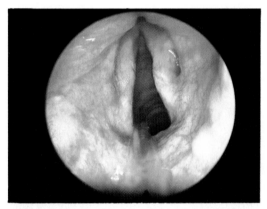
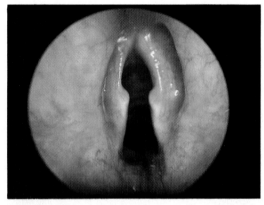

Figure 309. Chronic laryngitis in an adult with a persistently husky voice. Multiple biopsies showed nonspecific "dysplasia" but no evidence of atypia or of malignancy.

Figure 310. Very prominent arytenoids and vocal processes in a debilitated elderly man with a weak, breathy voice (so-called myasthenia laryngis).

REINKE'S EDEMA AND VOCAL CORD POLYPS

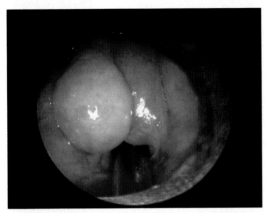

Figure 311. Huge bilateral polyps from neglected, untreated Reinke's edema.

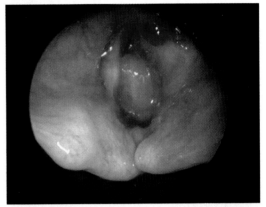

Figure 312. Same patient as in Figure 311. Site of the left polyp removed 4 weeks earlier has healed prior to removal of the pathology on the right side.

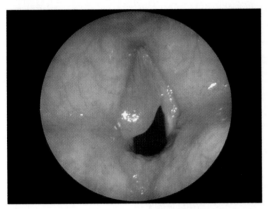

Figure 313. Polypoidal Reinke's edema on the left side. The right side had been treated 4 weeks before.

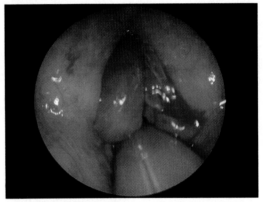

Figure 314. Gross bilateral vocal cord Reinke's edema. The airway was difficult to maintain during anesthesia, and an endotracheal tube that was passed caused some trauma and bleeding on the right side.

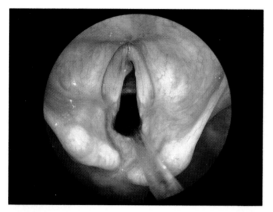

Figure 315. Small vocal cord polyp at the anterior end of the left vocal cord.

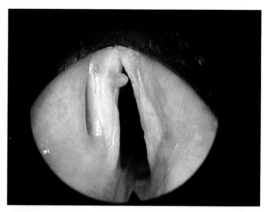

Figure 316. Small protruding vocal cord polyp on the left side.

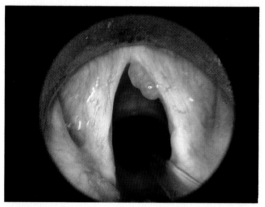

Figure 317. Soft, sessile polyp on the edge of the anterior third of the right vocal cord.

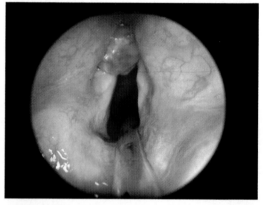

Figure 318. Large granular polyp, possibly an organized hematoma, at the anterior commissure on the left side.

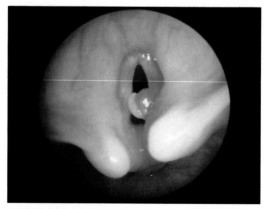

Figure 319. Posterior hemorrhagic polyp on the right side in an 8-year-old child who had suffered direct neck trauma 6 days before. An edematous organizing hematoma.

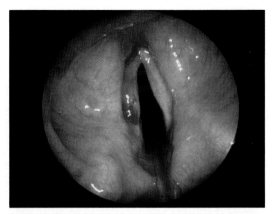

Figure 320. Polypoidal upper surface of the left vocal cord with some recent submucosal bleeding.

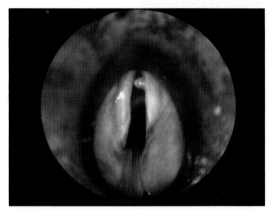

Figure 321. Small but firm polyp on the anterior edge of the right vocal cord. Reported as a pyogenic granuloma after histological examination, but probably an organized hematoma.

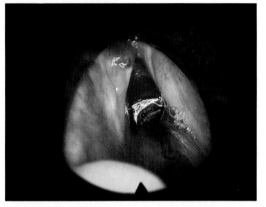

Figure 322. Large polyp on the left side.

VOCAL GRANULOMAS AND VOCAL ULCERS

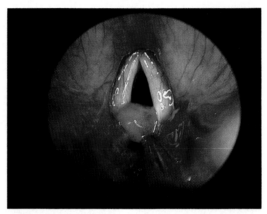

Figure 323. Moderate-sized left vocal granuloma arising from the typical site, the medial surface of the arytenoid cartilage.

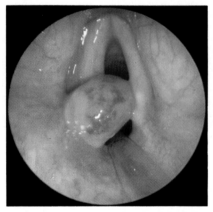 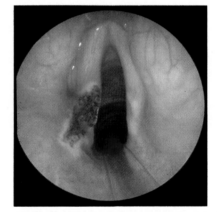

Figure 324. *A,* Large pale pink vocal granuloma. *B,* After removal using the carbon dioxide laser.

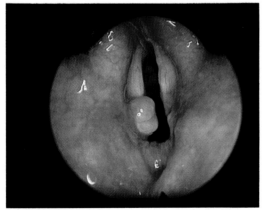 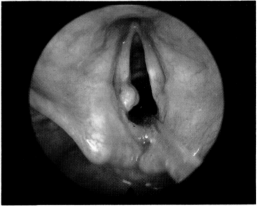

Figure 325. Small vocal granuloma arising near the left vocal process. The jet tube has been placed in the anterior commissure to give an unobstructed view.

Figure 326. Small left "hyperacidic" vocal cord granuloma in an adult patient with a hiatus hernia and gastroesophageal reflux.

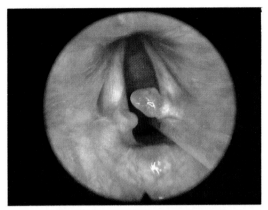

Figure 327. Bilateral intubation granuloma larger on the right than the left, 7 weeks after the causative intubation.

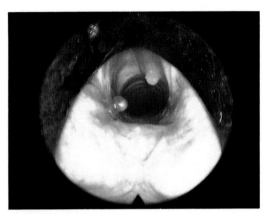

Figure 328. Small intubation granuloma in an atypical site, in the subglottic region posterior to and below the vocal process.

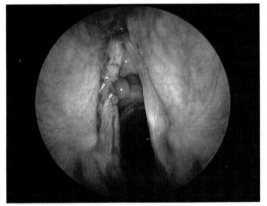

Figure 329. A rounded, edematous granuloma at the site of recent laser surgery. A "laser granuloma" occurs when carbon particles act as an irritative focus in the submucosal tissues.

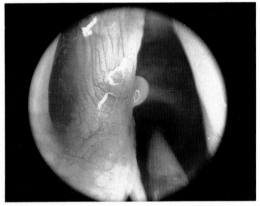

Figure 330. Close-up view of another "laser granuloma" 5 weeks after removal of papilloma from this site.

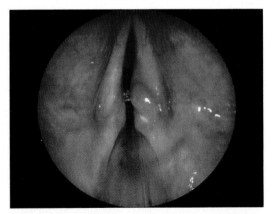

Figure 331. Bilateral vocal "ulcers" with pronounced surrounding edema on the right side. The edges of the ulcers actually show the histological changes of pachyderma.

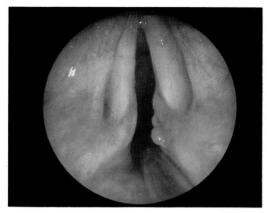

Figure 332. Right-sided vocal ulcer with an irregular base affecting the medial edge of the arytenoid posteriorly.

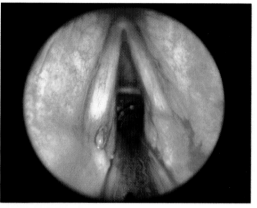

Figure 333. Bilateral vocal ulcers with fairly smooth, heaped-up edges.

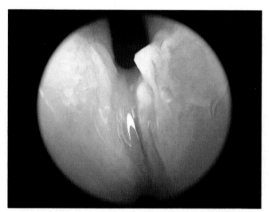

Figure 334. Acute ulcer in the posterior glottis on the right side. This was an incidental finding in a patient undergoing endoscopy for other reasons. Histopathological examination showed "acute ulcer," cause unknown.

MULTIPLE
RESPIRATORY
PAPILLOMATOSIS

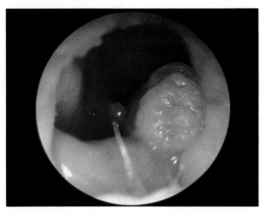

Figure 335. Mass of papilloma in one nasal cavity in a 14-year-old boy who had no other papillomas.

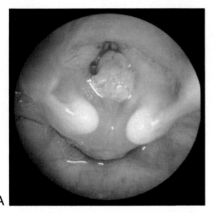

A

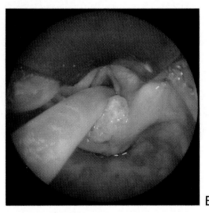

B

Figure 336. *A,* Pendunculated mass of papilloma above the vocal cords in a newborn baby. There was intermittent airway obstruction with cyanotic attacks. *B,* An endotracheal tube was necessary to secure and maintain the airway while the mass was removed.

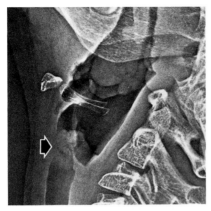

Figure 337. Papillomas above, at, and below the vocal cords (*arrow*), the site of predilection, seen clearly on the preliminary xerogram.

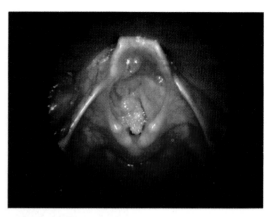

Figure 338. Endoscopy in a 7-year-old shows multiple papillomas, a large mass in the left hemilarynx, and scattered lesions on the posterior surface of the epiglottis. Facilities to pass an endotracheal tube or a bronchoscope must be readily at hand during induction of anesthesia.

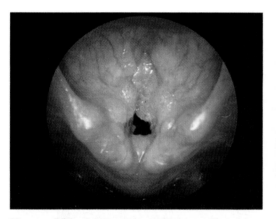

Figure 339. Adult with multiple papillomas on the true and false vocal cords on each side and moderately severe respiratory obstruction.

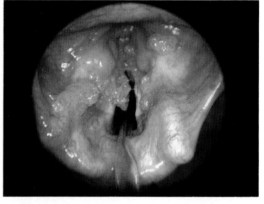

Figure 340. Widely scattered papillomas, worse on the left side but with some normal vocal cord edges seen.

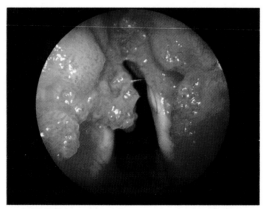

Figure 341. Close-up view of the papillomas seen in Figure 340, showing the typical appearance.

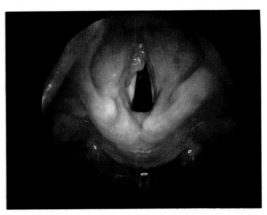

Figure 342. Small mass of papilloma from the anterior aspect of the left ventricle in an adult male. It may be necessary to bounce the laser beam from a metal mirror or to use angled cupped forceps.

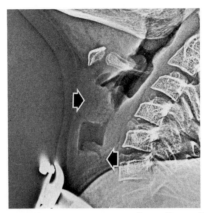

Figure 343. Huge masses of papilloma in the larynx at and above the tracheotomy tube (upper arrow) in a 7-year-old child. When the child was 18 months of age, the papillomas were diagnosed and a tracheotomy was performed. Papillomas have proliferated at the tracheotomy site (lower arrow).

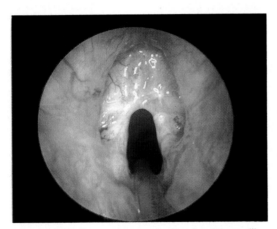

Figure 344. Large postsurgical web with papillomas on the upper surface of the web and on the vocal cords posteriorly.

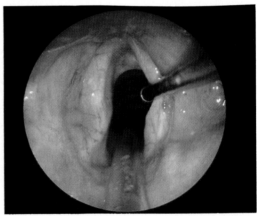

Figure 345. Small anterior subglottic web following previous papilloma surgery. The web can be seen only at direct laryngoscopy performed with the patient under general anesthesia.

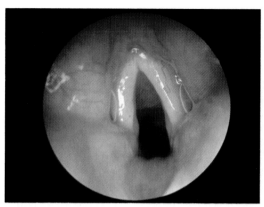

Figure 346. Larynx of a patient who has had nine laser treatments for laryngeal papillomas. There is no web or scarring, but there is slight edema with rounding of the edge of each vocal fold.

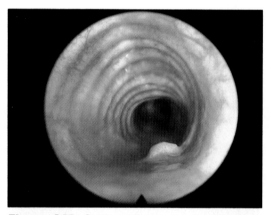

Figure 347. Small papilloma on the posterior wall of the upper trachea in a patient with laryngeal papillomas.

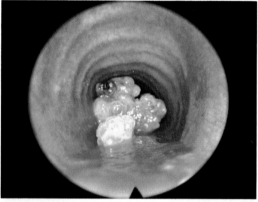

Figure 348. Large mass of papilloma in the mid-trachea in a 28-year-old man who presented with noisy breathing. There were no other papillomas.

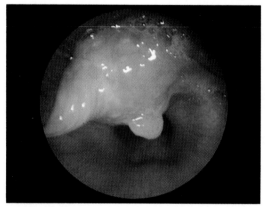

Figure 349. Small mass of papilloma in the postcricoid region on the right. Laryngeal papillomas also present.

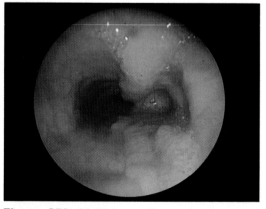

Figure 350. Multiple papillomas in the upper third of the esophagus in a patient with multiple respiratory papillomatosis. Such lesions are uncommon in the esophagus.

CYSTIC DISEASE IN THE LARYNX

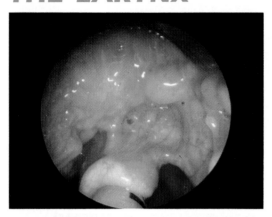

Figure 351. Small ductal retention cyst in the right vallecula in a child.

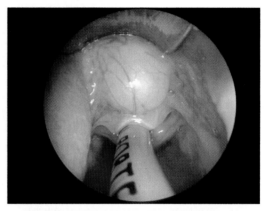

Figure 352. Thyroglossal duct cyst in an infant. It is in the midline at the base of the tongue at the foramen cecum.

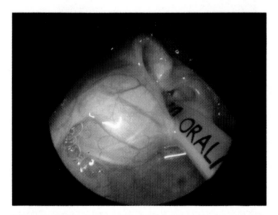

Figure 353. Large ductal retention cyst in the left supraglottic hemilarynx of an infant. There was severe stridor, and a rounded cystic mass could be seen on a lateral x-ray.

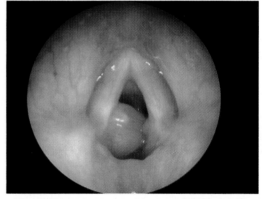

Figure 354. Ductal retention cyst almost filling the subglottic region in an infant. There was a second cyst below. The cysts were diagnosed and treated by endoscopic means.

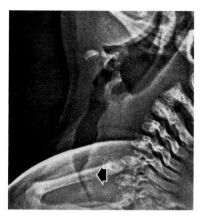

Figure 355. Severe narrowing of the upper tracheal lumen (*arrow*) by a rounded mass arising from the posterior tracheal wall.

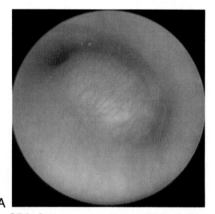
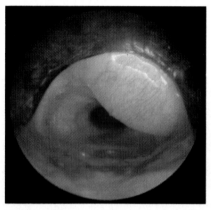

A
B

Figure 356. Same case as Figure 355. *A,* Tracheoscopy shows severe obstruction of the lumen by a cystic mass on the left posterolateral wall. *B,* Esophagoscopy shows a rounded cystic mass from the right anterolateral wall. The lesion was a rare duplication cyst of the trachea.

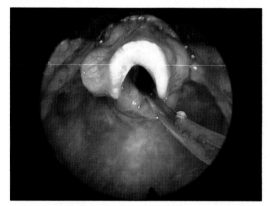
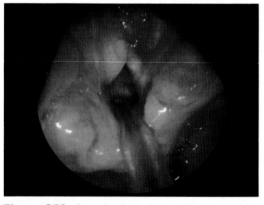

Figure 357. Ductal retention cyst on the lateral aspect of the epiglottis in an adult. It was causing no symptoms.

Figure 358. Anterior lateral saccular cyst on the left side in a 10-year-old girl. This is a mucous-filled internal laryngocele arising from the saccule at the anterior end of the ventricle.

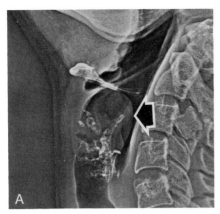
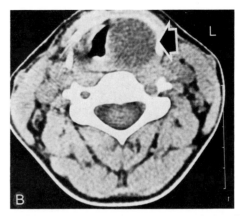

Figure 359. Large cystic lesion in a 20-year-old woman seen (*A*) on the lateral xerogram (*arrow*), and (*B*) on the CT scan (*arrow*). It is in the left supraglottic region and is causing partial airway obstruction.

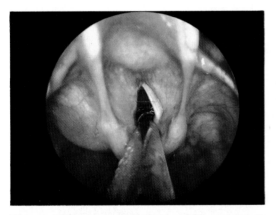
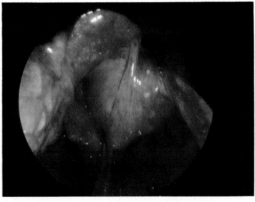

Figure 360. The cyst in Figure 359 as seen at endoscopy. It was removed with the laser and proved to be a rare developmental cyst of the internal perichondrium lining the thyroid cartilage.

Figure 361. Large right supraglottic lateral saccular cyst in a 73-year-old woman with slight huskiness and a muffled voice. No other pathology was found in the larynx, and the lesion was successfully removed with the laser.

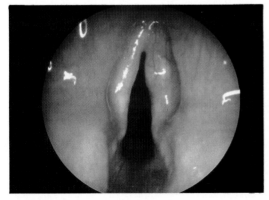
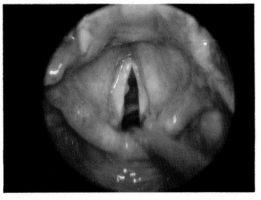

Figure 362. Intracordal cyst in the right vocal cord with some minor reactive changes in the left vocal cord.

Figure 363. Small but prominent ductal retention cyst of a mucous gland on the left vocal cord in a 35-year-old man.

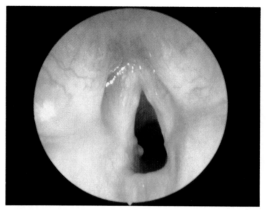

Figure 364. Two small posteriorly placed ductal retention cysts following previous prolonged intubation in a 3-year-old patient.

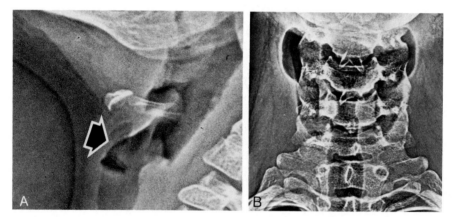

Figure 365. *A,* A normal air-filled laryngeal saccule (*arrow*) is sometimes seen on a radiograph. The ventricle of the larynx is seen with the true cords below it and the false cords above. *B,* An 18-year-old trumpet player with bilateral air-filled laryngoceles in the neck seen on an anteroposterior xerogram.

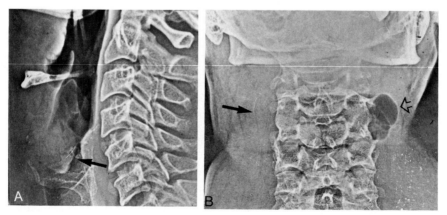

Figure 366. *A,* The lateral xerogram in a 28-year-old man with mild huskiness and intermittent breathing obstruction shows a more-or-less rounded opacity in the larynx (*arrow*). *B,* The anteroposterior xerogram shows an air-filled laryngocele in the left neck (*open arrow*) and confirms a laryngomucocele on the right side (*closed arrow*). The latter was removed surgically.

VOCAL CORD PARALYSIS AND INJECTION OF TEFLON

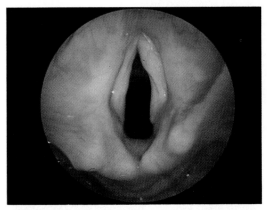

Figure 367. Right vocal cord paralysis in a 5-year-old child with a weak cry since birth.

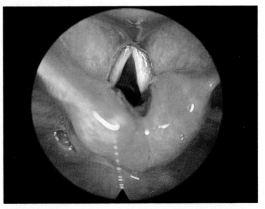

Figure 368. Left vocal cord paralysis in an adolescent.

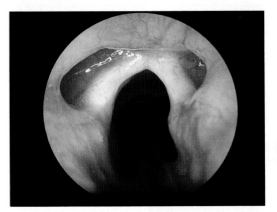

Figure 369. Short and immobile right vocal cord in a 16-year-old who had a weak, breathy voice. The glottic opening is of unusual shape. There were associated abnormalities of cranial nerves IX and XI on the right side. Probable congenital anomaly of the brain stem nuclei.

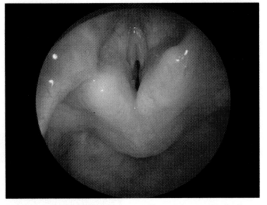

Figure 370. Bilateral vocal cord paralysis in a 3-year-old child.

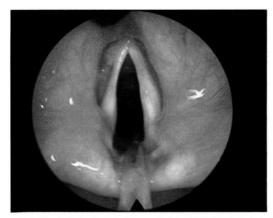

Figure 371. Left vocal cord paralyzed for 18 years since cardiac surgery. The left cord is thin and atrophic.

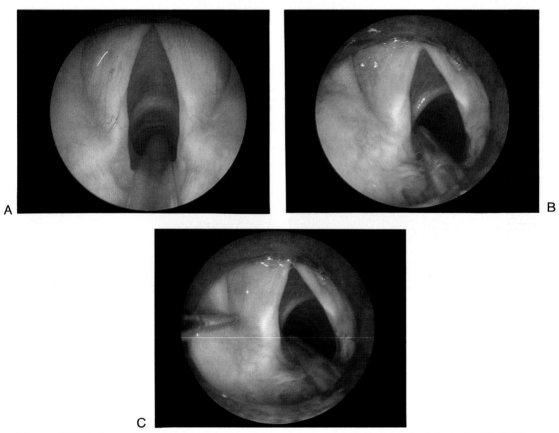

Figure 372. Left vocal cord paralysis in an adult man. The cord is about to be injected with Gelfoam paste. *A,* The larynx has been exposed and the jet anesthesia tube is in the posterior commissure. *B,* The left false cord has been pushed aside to expose the floor and lateral aspect of the left laryngeal ventricle. *C,* The 19-gauge needle of the injection "gun" is introduced as far laterally as possible to deliver the paste.

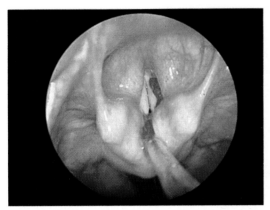

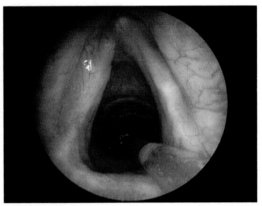

Figure 373. Closure of the left vocal cord after completion of injection of the right hemilarynx. As vocal cord movement returns, the adequacy of the filling can be judged.

Figure 374. Teflon has been injected into the left vocal cord many months before but with no improvement of the voice. The injection has been wrongly placed in the membranous cord, not posterior and lateral to the vocal process of the arytenoid.

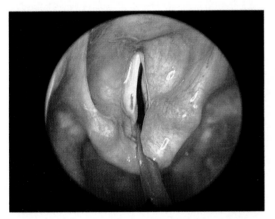

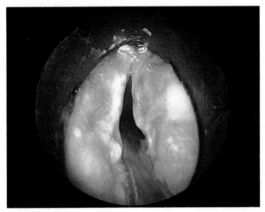

Figure 375. The right side has been previously injected with too much Teflon, resulting in a poor voice. The right hemilarynx is overfull, and the vocal cord cannot be seen. It is very difficult to reverse this problem.

Figure 376. Granulomatous reaction, possibly related to prior cytotoxic treatment for lymphoma, in a man who had previously had Teflon injected into the right vocal cord.

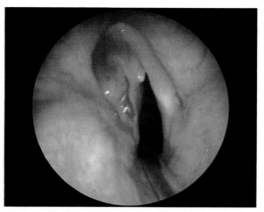

Figure 377. Grossly distorted left hemilarynx following previous injection of too much Teflon too superficially. Most of it was painstakingly removed with the laser, but the hemilarynx became scarred and the voice result was very poor.

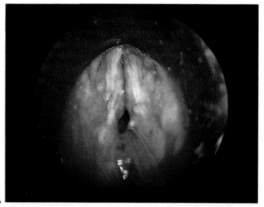
A

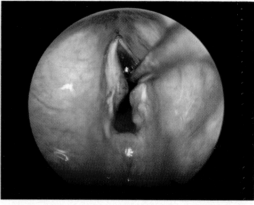
B

Figure 378. A middle-aged woman who had been given two injections of Teflon in one vocal cord and one injection in the other vocal cord had severe stridor and airway obstruction at rest. *A,* Both vocal cords have been overinjected with Teflon; there was movement in each side. A tracheotomy was necessary. *B,* Two weeks after the tracheotomy, there are left and right subglottic masses due to misplaced Teflon. Large amounts of Teflon were removed on each side and the tracheotomy was removed, but the voice remained very poor.

EPITHELIAL DYSPLASIA AND MALIGNANCY

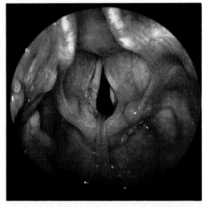 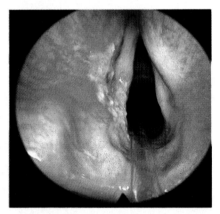

Figure 379. Severe epithelial dysplasia in the posterior part of the left side of the larynx on the true cord and false cord in a 70-year-old man. The anterior end of the right false cord partly obscures the left vocal fold.

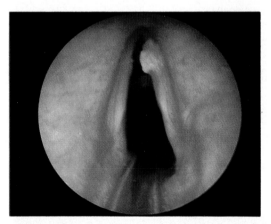 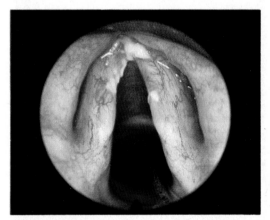

Figure 380. Raised area of leukoplakia at the anterior end of the right false cord. Histologically this was shown to be hyperkeratosis without atypia.

Figure 381. Scattered areas of leukoplakia in a 67-year-old heavy smoker. Biopsy showed epithelial dysplasia but no atypia.

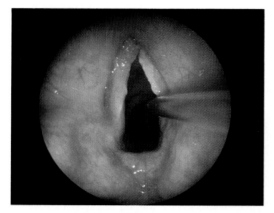

Figure 382. Papilloma and dyskeratosis on the anterior end of the left vocal cord and hyperkeratosis on the right side in a 48-year-old woman on immunosuppressants following a renal transplant.

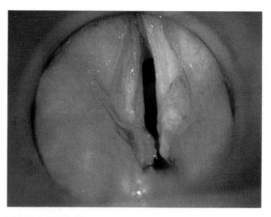

Figure 383. Chronic mucosal changes on the left side, less on the right. Repeated biopsies showed hyperkeratosis with atypia but no malignancy.

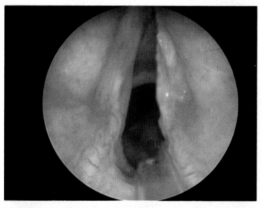

Figure 384. The left vocal cord of a 58-year-old man was treated with the defocused laser beam 4 weeks earlier for hyperkeratosis with atypia. The right side is about to be similarly treated.

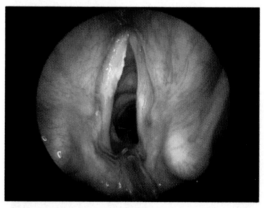

Figure 385. The white area on the anterior half of the left vocal cord was found histologically to be acanthosis.

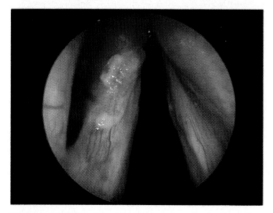

Figure 386. Noninvasive carcinoma-in-situ. View with a 50° angled telescope showing leukoplakia and a raised irregular area on the anterior half of the left vocal cord. Laser treatment was used for this lesion.

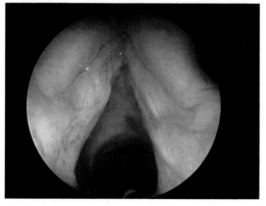

Figure 387. Carcinoma-in-situ of the left vocal cord in a 56-year-old man.

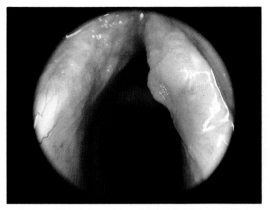

Figure 388. Bilateral epithelial irregularity. Biopsies of both sides showed carcinoma-in-situ. Staged laser treatment was employed.

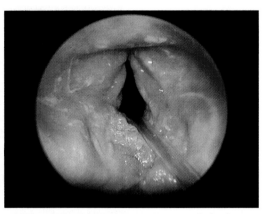

Figure 389. Verrucous carcinoma of the larynx in a 62-year-old man treated with the laser.

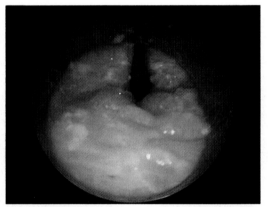

Figure 390. Verrucous carcinoma of the posterior larynx in a 61-year-old woman, which was successfully controlled with repeated laser treatments.

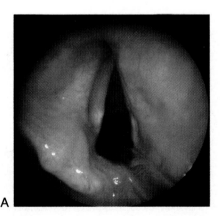

A

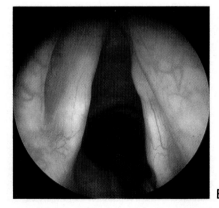

B

Figure 391. *A,* The right vocal cord cannot be seen until the laryngoscope is introduced further. *B,* A finely granular rounded mass in the center of the right membranous cord was a small invasive carcinoma.

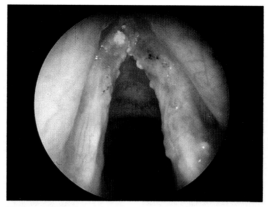

Figure 392. Invasive squamous cell carcinoma of the right vocal cord, anterior commissure, and anterior end of the left vocal cord. The patient was treated with radiotherapy.

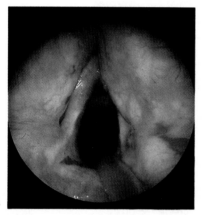

A

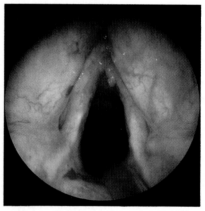

B

Figure 393. *A,* Overhang obscuring anterior end of the right vocal cord. *B,* Small invasive squamous cell carcinoma on the anterior end of the right vocal cord near the anterior commissure. The treatment used was partial laryngectomy conservation surgery.

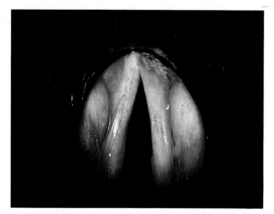

Figure 394. Final result after radiation therapy for an invasive squamous cell carcinoma that was in the anterior end of the left laryngeal ventricle.

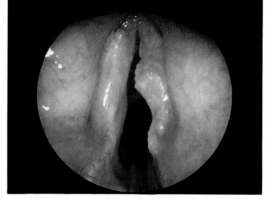

Figure 395. Invasive squamous cell carcinoma in the right vocal cord. There was good movement of the cord. Radiotherapy was the treatment used.

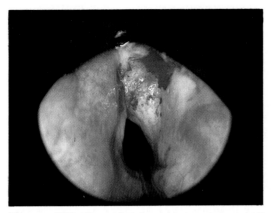

Figure 396. Extensive invasive squamous cell carcinoma of the right vocal cord, which was immobile. There were no metastases to regional lymph nodes. Radiotherapy was employed.

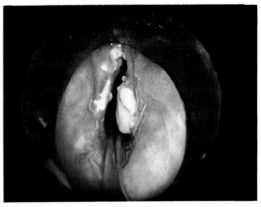

Figure 397. The gross appearance suggests the possibility of a granuloma of the right vocal cord and severe changes in the remainder of the epithelium. The large right lesion was a squamous cell carcinoma, and on the left side there was epithelial dysplasia. The patient was treated with radiotherapy.

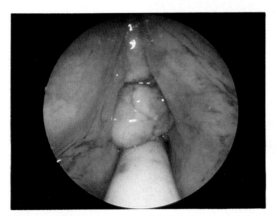

Figure 398. Large mass of infiltrating squamous cell carcinoma in the left vocal cord with regional metastases in the neck. Laryngectomy and neck dissection were necessary.

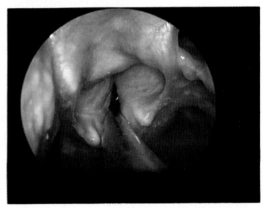

Figure 399. Squamous cell carcinoma in the right hemilarynx with intact mucous membrane in a 67-year-old smoker with a husky voice. Direct laryngoscopy showed a fullness in the right hemilarynx. Laser incision through the intact mucous membrane and deep biopsy with cupped forceps gave a positive frozen-section biopsy.

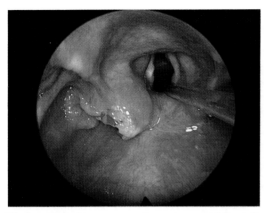

Figure 400. Squamous cell carcinoma of the left piriform fossa extending to the lateral surface of the arytenoid.

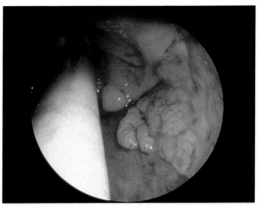

Figure 401. Large infiltrating squamous cell carcinoma of the right lateral pharyngeal wall.

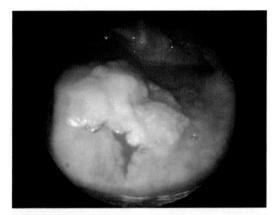

Figure 402. Infiltrating squamous cell carcinoma on the posterior pharyngeal wall. A large ulcer with a sloughing surface that bled easily when touched.

RARE AND UNUSUAL CONDITIONS

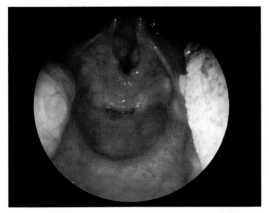

Figure 403. An apparent semicircular web in the posterior pharyngeal wall in an infant, but probably a normal variant.

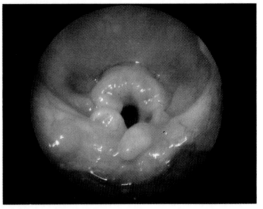

Figure 404. Congenital hypoplasia of the epiglottis, aryepiglottic folds, and arytenoids in a child with stridor and a tendency toward aspiration.

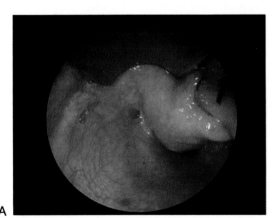

A

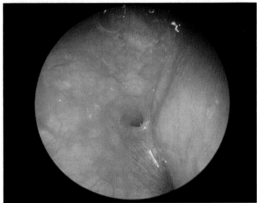

B

Figure 405. *A,* Opening of a fourth branchial pouch in the left piriform fossa in a 4-month-old infant with severe stridor and a swelling in the neck and upper mediastinum due to infection in the pouch. *B,* Close-up view of same opening.

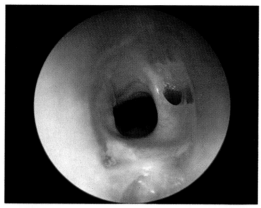

Figure 406. A blind sinus in the immediate subglottic region on the right in a 3-month-old infant with intermittent stridor. An attenuated form of duplication of the trachea.

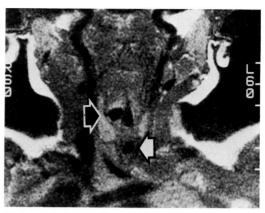

Figure 407. MRI showing a tracheotomy opening (*white arrow*). On the right of the air-filled subglottic region there is a rounded air-filled cyst (*black arrow*).

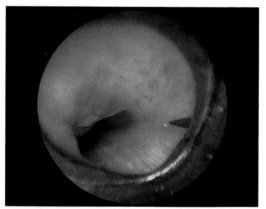

Figure 408. Same case as in Figure 406. There is narrowing of the subglottic airway and a slitlike opening on the right, held open by the end of the bronchoscope. At operation a congenital cyst involving the cricoid cartilage was removed.

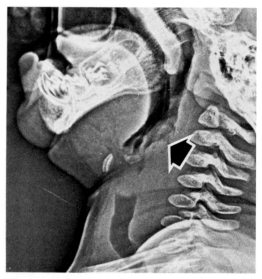

Figure 409. Irregular mass (*arrow*) on the posterior wall of the laryngopharynx in a 6-week-old baby with stridor, difficulty feeding, and failure to thrive.

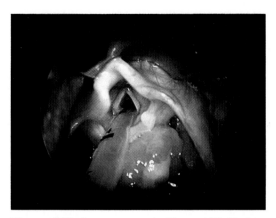

Figure 410. Same case as in Figure 409. Endoscopy reveals an irregular mass behind the larynx, arising from the posterior pharyngeal wall. It is a choristoma consisting of ectopic gastric mucosa. Laser removal was followed by complete resolution of symptoms.

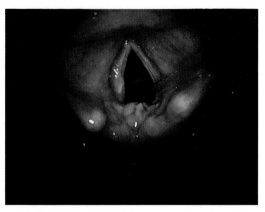

Figure 411. Pachyonychia congenita in the posterior commissure of a 14-year-old boy. A very rare laryngeal manifestation of a rare skin condition.

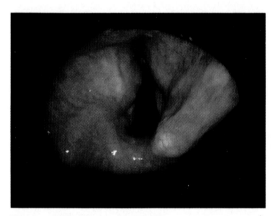

Figure 412. Bilateral neurofibromas, one on each side of the supraglottic larynx.

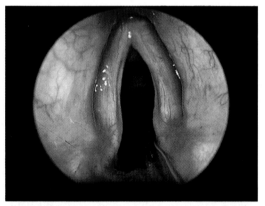

Figure 413. Bilateral vocal sulcus, so-called duplication of the vocal cord, causing minimal effect on the voice quality.

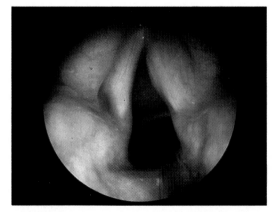

Figure 414. A lymphosarcoma in the right vocal cord with intact mucosa. The first clinical manifestation of this generalized disease was progressive huskiness.

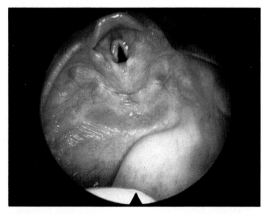

Figure 415. Right parapharyngeal neurofibroma in an infant. Smooth mass in the nasopharyngeal wall presenting below the soft palate.

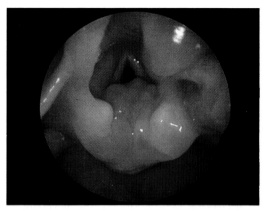

Figure 416. Endoscopic view showed a raised irregular midline granuloma in the posterior commissure. Findings of repeated biopsy over several years have been nonspecific, and the cause is unknown.

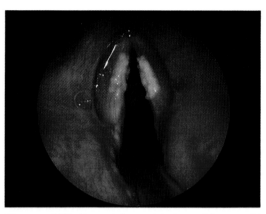

Figure 417. Fungal laryngitis in a 14-year-old boy with asthma, related to long-term inhalation of a metered aerosol steroid spray.

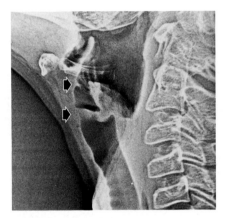

Figure 418. Supraglottic (*upper arrow*) and glottic (*lower arrow*) webbing in a 10-year-old with epidermolysis bullosa.

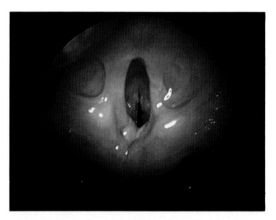

Figure 419. The supraglottic and glottic webbing can be seen at endoscopy, which must be done with great care so as not to provoke any further mucosal reaction in an already compromised airway.

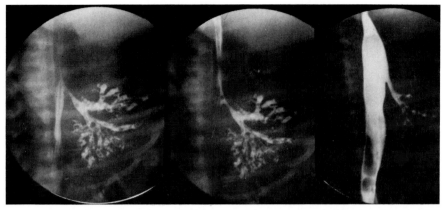

Figure 420. A pulmonary segment arising from the esophagus is visible on contrast esophagography.

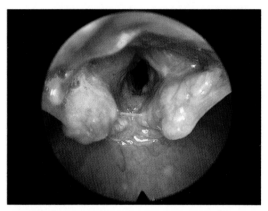

Figure 421. Primary amyloid deposits in the supraglottic, glottic, and subglottic larynx in a 37-year-old woman with slowly progressive hoarseness and weakness of the voice over 6 or 7 years.

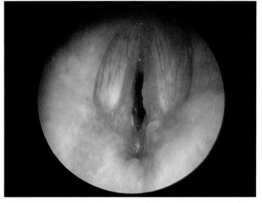

Figure 422. Primary amyloid deposits in the subglottic tissues on each side in a 32-year-old woman. Preliminary tracheotomy was performed, and repeated laser treatments later allowed the tracheotomy to be removed.

Index

Note: Page numbers in *italics* refer to illustrations.

171